W9-CDK-955

CHILDREN'S SPEECH

Under the advisory editorship of
J. JEFFERY AUER

CHILDREN'S SPEECH:

a practical introduction to communication development

ROBERT HOPPER
University of Texas

RITA C. NAREMORE
Indiana University

HARPER & ROW, Publishers

New York, Evanston, San Francisco, London

To Brian and Jay

If they could tell us, they would let us know

CONTENTS

PREFACE

HOW TO READ THIS BOOK

When a social scientist says something that cannot be understood by a relatively intelligent seventh-grader, someone is jiving someone.

Neil Postman and Charles Weingartner,
The Soft Revolution

Though we expect few seventh graders to read this book, our aim has been to say things simply enough so that readers with little or no background in the social sciences will not be inundated by technical terms and abstract theory. With this in mind, we have tried to do three things:

1. *Write simply.* We have tried to use everyday English, avoiding technical terms except where they are absolutely necessary. Where technical terms appear, we have tried to define them, or to give an example of what we mean.

2. *Put citations in parentheses.* Rather than using footnotes, we cite sources from whom we have borrowed material by putting the author's last name and the date of the publication in parentheses right in the text: Smith, 1968. Simply ignore these citations unless you want to read further on the subject, then look up the full citation in the list of references at the end of the book.

3. *List some readings at the end of each chapter.* At the end of each chapter is a section called "Read This." In it are several books and articles on the topic discussed in the chapter, along with some notes about which ones will be most helpful to you.

Like all "current and relevant" teaching materials, this book has a behavioral objective: to inspire you to read one of the

"Read This" selections for each chapter. Only when you do that will you understand the complex fascination that the field of communication development holds for so many students, researchers, and teachers.

We wish to acknowledge the patience of the families and colleagues who tolerated us and helped us as we wrote this book. Especially, we recognize our debt to mentor-friend Fred Williams. He didn't teach us all we know about children, but he showed us how to still speak plainly even when mesmerized by research ideas.

ROBERT HOPPER
RITA C. NAREMORE

PART ONE

chapter 1

THE CHILD'S GARDEN
OF ELOQUENCE

Children's communication development attracts widespread attention these days—for many good reasons. Recent research has brought startling advances in what we know about children's speech, language, and learning abilities.

Teachers welcome these new insights because only with such information can schools be made more effective and humane places. These advances are no less relevant to therapists and clinicians. As we learn more about normal communication development, we can define better what is not normal—which improves prospects for therapeutic treatment of children with speech or emotional handicaps. And, of course, parents also are concerned because their children must learn so many communication skills in the preschool years. Finally, it can be argued that all Americans should be aware of research in this area. If the "American dream"—a just society in which there is equality of opportunity for all citizens—is to be realized, we must know how to help all children learn better and perhaps even more important, communicate more effectively.

Important as these goals are, there are other reasons for being fascinated by how children communicate. It's not just that "kids say the darndest things"—although Art Linkletter and any parent will tell you they do. Young children also exhibit a vivacity in communicating and learning that can serve as a model for everyone. Whatever the stuff of life is, children have an overflow supply. Just watch a group of four-year-olds play—they *always* run.

The same boundless energy and creativity children show in playing tag is unleashed in the more important task-game of learning to communicate. We say task-game because parents and teachers take it more seriously than the children do. Kids are most interested (and probably learn most) while playing. Listen to a two-year-old in his crib waiting for sleep, or a three-year-old playing alone with her dolls. Children play with sounds, with putting words together to create and re-create events of the day. They create because the act of creation seems to be a delightful experience. Here is a monologue spoken by two-and-a-half-year-old Brian Hopper, playing in the bathtub.

> Chim chiminey chiminey
> Chim chiminey chiminey
> Here come some
> I be right there
> I want someone to wash me
> wiff my wash cloff
> washy washy cloth
> I got it all full (referring to washcloth, which he put in mouth,
>   then spat several times)
>
> No
> Well, hard
> Chim chiminey chiminey
> Chiminey
> I love you
>
> With that
> At the other page, she can get it
> A store
> An hour, an' a page
> (in falsetto) Honey, can't wash me
> No no, and we let it out
> And she doesn't want me to remember you
> Washy washy
> Oh the bizzin of the bees (alteration of "Big Rock Candy Moun-
>   tain")
> Oh the bizzin of the bees

Oh the bizzin of the bees
Oh the bizzin of the bees
Oh the bizzin of the bees
Mix mix mix
Don't like that water
Chim chiminey, I'll poo soo
Chim chiminey
Some more
(pause)

Oh the bizzin a the bees
Oh the bizzin a the bees
Oh the bizzin of the bees
Oh the bizzin a the bees
2, 3, 4, 5, 6, 7 (with melodious emphasis) you guys
Would you like my boat?
(several unintelligible sounds) some more
I think that's about enough
Now let's put my washcloth in

Chim chiminey
Mix
Mix a orange juice
It's a washy
Now
Wait to see what she
Oh, happy, really

Chim chiminey chiminey
Hey chiminey boy
Hey, four como
Hey chiminey chiminey
Um (pause)

Hey, Mommy
I already called

While the child plays in this fashion, he learns to speak his native language. And a language is a lot to learn. Imagine how you would feel if you woke up one morning and found yourself in some strange culture where everybody spoke a language you did not understand. Adults (especially those who teach) would be overwhelmed by the enormity of what they would have to learn in order to communicate. Yet this is exactly what little children succeed in learning long before school age, usually with no formal instruction. And, as shown by the above example, they usually have a great time doing it.

We must point out, lest we be accused of taking too narrow a view, that we are both parents and thus have learned that children are beastly and unpleasant just as often as they are cute and angelic. But regardless of how an adult may feel about any single child at any given moment, the world of his speech permits them to look at a part of youth just barely beyond their memory. Children's speech reveals a great deal about how people learn, how people motivate themselves, how people create, and more.

A child speaking is an esthetic event. It is also both educational and rhetorical-persuasive in nature. Through learning to talk, children learn how to do well in society. And as they learn, they create beauty. The samples of child speech you will read in the following chapters are cut flowers from the child's garden of eloquence.

WHERE WE ARE GOING

The goal of this book is to explain how children learn to talk.

First, children's speech must be considered as a biological event. Man's unique heritage is to be the speaking animal. Children talk as naturally as they stand up to walk, and almost as naturally as they grow toenails and baby fat. In Chapter 2 communication development is examined in the context of nonhuman communication systems and man's unique biological endowment.

Second, various aspects of the act of learning to talk must be analyzed. In one sense, acquisition of speaking ability is a single developmental matrix of events. In another, it is a collection of specific aspects of development—each aspect having its own history, and each spawning a group of scientists who study only it. Part Two summarizes significant research in several areas: development of the sound system (Chapter 3), development of syntax (Chapter 4), development of semantics (Chapter 5), and development of pragmatics (Chapter 6). Chapter 7 considers the impact of communication development upon development of thinking, and vice versa.

Third, the eternal scholarly questions must be raised: How can all this information be synthesized? How can it be used to bring us closer to the American dream? These issues are discussed in Part Three. An attempt is made in Chapter 8 to put the entire matrix of communicative development back together again —a task not unlike that faced by all the king's horses and all the king's men. Chapters 9, 10, and 11 apply this information to current educational problems, to communication patterns of minority-group children, and to problems of speech and language therapy.

chapter 2

CHILD SPEECH AS A BIOLOGICAL PROCESS

Children's communication development is considered in terms of biology because a child's talk is as much a part of his natural development as his growing two sets of teeth. Some biological concepts have interesting applications to human communication development, and it is also informative to view the process of learning to talk in light of nonhuman communication systems in nature.

DIFFERENTIATION

Each of us begins life as a single-celled organism, or zygote, which then reproduces itself. After a while there is a small collection of cells, each of which is precisely like the original cell. (Think of a handful of marbles.) Some of the cells are inside the group, others are on the outside. Due to the influences of these different surroundings, inside cells and outside cells become less alike. So begins the process called *differentiation*. There is no complete explanation for differentiation. It simply is the process in which things start out alike, but end up dissimilar. A human embryo starts out as one cell that multiplies to produce millions of cells of many varieties. Some cells "specialize" to make blood, others to constitute tooth enamel, and so forth. The types of cells that develop in a growing person are not a matter of chance. As zygotes, you and I were already coded to be people. Further, our genetic structures specified our eye color, skin color, and general range of intelligence. We inherited these genetic structures from our ancestors.

Just as certain physical characteristics are genetically coded, certain behaviors are also a result of heredity. Such hereditary, or innate, behaviors are often called *instinctive*. Baby ducks, for example, follow moving objects the size of their mothers; this behavior seems to be genetically determined, just as are physical characteristics such as the structure of the duck's webbed feet. Each species of animals performs certain unique and inherited behaviors: Dogs bark, spiders spin intricate webs, and birds go through elaborate courtship rituals. In the sense that webs are unique to spiders, human language appears to be unique to people.

The relationship between our biological heritage and our language behavior will be discussed throughout this book. For example, some aspects of communication development unfold in a manner that recalls the differentiation of complicated life forms from single-celled zygotes. Similar processes of differentiation can be seen in the development of language structure (syntax), the sound system (phonology), and the meaning system (semantics). The concept is introduced at this point to indicate that the capacity and the process of learning to communicate, even in structural form, resembles the growth of life itself.

The differentiation of speech and language forms is unique to man, but many other animals communicate. Examining human communication in light of other communication systems in nature reveals further information about child speech as a biological process.

COMMUNICATION IN NATURE

Although man is not the only communicator, his language is the most impressively complex one which has been discovered. These are some things human communicators can do:

1. *Express emotions.* By shifting the physical quality of his voice, man can express varied emotional states. When the pretty blonde being murdered in the horror movie screams, we know that she is communicating terror. When the teenager watching the

movie whispers sweet nothings in his girl friend's ear, his emotions are also readily understandable. Even babies can express emotions—they can let us know how they feel long before they can talk. As we grow, we learn to use language to express more precise emotions.

2. *Refer to and describe events and objects.* Man can point out and describe anything from a tree to tranquility because human language assigns arbitrary fixed meanings to words and constructions—meanings that have no necessary connection with the objects to which they refer. This makes description an easy task once the code is learned. Many of the child's first sentences are descriptive: "Red truck," "Ball all gone," "Big tree."

3. *Combine sounds into complicated structures,* with each structure (phrase or sentence) being a meaningful unit. Man's capacity for syntax, which is probably his most remarkable communication ability, will be discussed in Chapter 4. At this point we note only that sentences are very complex structures, and the learning of these structures by children is a major aspect of their communication development.

Each of these abilities is used many times each day. This capacity is a result of our being the only creatures who can do all three of these things. Yet no one of these abilities is unique to man; each exists in some form in nature. All mammals can express emotion. The typical American dog is easily understandable when he growls at the postman, whines to be let outside, or barks happily at other dogs. Description of environment also occurs among nonpeople. The best example is the well-known "dance of the bees": Bees that have found food dance around the hive to describe to other bees the distance and direction of the food source. Man's ability to combine smaller units into larger ones to obtain more complex meanings also has parallels in nature. Some birds, for example, combine smaller song segments into larger ones in a manner similar to man's combining of sounds and phrases into sentences.

MONKEY SEE, MONKEY DO?

The whole question of how animals communicate has led some researchers to ask whether human language can be taught to nonhumans. Because apes are closer to man on the evolutionary ladder than any other animal, they have been the subjects of the most interesting of these teaching experiments. Most attempts to teach language to apes have been undertaken within the framework of learning theory, on the premise that lower forms of life might learn higher systems with carefully administered reinforcement. If all such attempts fail, then evidence mounts that language is unique to man.

Early experimenters tried to get apes to make human sounds. With their failure, interest in ape speech declined. Recently, however, two sets of researchers have attempted to teach chimpanzees linguistic behavior in the form of sign languages.

Premack (1971) taught a chimpanzee to use plastic symbols as words, and Gardner and Gardner (1969) taught their chimpanzee to use deaf sign language. Both apes have far outperformed their "cousins" in earlier experiments. Each has a relatively large vocabulary and can perform a variety of tasks—for example, answering questions. Neither, however, employs complex syntax or asks spontaneous "why" questions, as all little children do. The probable conclusion (although data from these experiments are still incomplete) is that language is the unique property of the human race.

GROWING UP COMMUNICATING

Just as communication patterns developed in early man, they develop in each growing child. The ways that his development shows itself demonstrate further that using language to communicate is a natural consequence of being human. Think about the shape of a person's mouth and throat, for instance. Language sounds are usually classified according to the positions of the articulators (tongue, teeth, etc.) when a sound is made. It would be difficult for other animals, whose mouths are very different from ours, to make these sounds. Early experiments to teach monkeys to talk failed partly because their mouths are shaped badly for speaking human languages.

Almost all children speak. We expect it of them, and classify them as abnormal if they fail to do so. We expect children who are exposed to language to speak regardless of the environment in which they are raised. If a child's parents are deaf and dumb, but he is physiologically normal, he will learn how to speak like any other child when he is exposed to language. And children do not seem to need much practice to learn to talk. Although the sounds babies make, particularly in the "babbling" stage, suggest speaking practice, this "practice" is of little help in learning to talk. Children who seldom babble still speak just as well as those who babble a great deal. Lenneberg (1966) reported the case of a fourteen-month-old child who had been unable to make any sounds for six months because of a throat operation. The day after his throat was repaired, the child made sounds typical of his age group without having babbled. No practice was required.

Finally, to some extent the development of communication seems to follow a regular schedule. Table 1 indicates how the development of communication skills parallels very closely the development of motor abilities. For example, at about age four months, the child coos and chuckles and, while sitting, is able to support his head. We caution you not to take literally the exact ages for the emergence of particular behaviors listed in the table. Children are not trains; they do not run on regular schedules. A child is not retarded if he does not coo until six months. The important point is that at about the same time that he coos, he will be able to support his head. Both seem to result from growth in the brain and nervous system.

In summary, all normal children learn to talk in similar ways and along similar schedules, with practice apparently having little importance. The only conclusion possible is that communicative development is closely tied to the general biological development of the human animal.

Inasmuch as the process of learning how to talk is the same for all people, what accounts for the uniqueness of each language? It is true that languages sound very different from each other. But there are also ways in which all languages are the same. Aspects of grammar that appear in all are called *linguistic universals*. Several linguistic universals have been discovered in the area of sound systems: All languages recognize a difference between vowels and consonants and all use syllables. Although no two languages are made up of identical sets of sounds, there does seem to be one large set of sounds from which all languages draw subsets. This set of sounds is best classified in terms of places of articulation in the human mouth. These issues will be discussed in Chapter 3.

There are also linguistic universals in the area of sentence structure (syntax): All languages have structural categories corresponding to noun phrase, verb phrase, and object. All languages construct sentences by showing grammatical relationships among these basic categories, but the way in which the relationships are established varies. In English, for example, most relationships between parts of sentences are shown through word order, but in Russian they are indicated by word endings—and word order is not highly constrained.

The existence of linguistic universals is further evidence that people are born with a capacity to learn language. These universals might be something that people simply know without being taught, just as a bird knows how to fly (instinctively). If you are a small child and if you instinctively know about language universals, all you need to learn is how speakers of your language represent those principles. Some scholars feel, for example, that the child innately knows about the relationship between subject and predicate in a sentence. Thus he needs to learn only that in English this relationship is expressed through word order. Whatever the form of the child's knowledge about language, it cannot be denied that humans are born with unique capacities for learning to speak.

WHAT DIFFERENCE DOES ENVIRONMENT MAKE?

At this point, you are probably ready to ask: If human communication is innate—that is, if children will talk no matter what we do—why should we worry so much about how parents and educators teach language skills to our children? You may also be seized by a feeling of helplessness: "If that's the way it is, there is no way we can improve things for our children."

Don't despair. How we teach our children *does* make a difference.

table 1
SIMULTANEOUS DEVELOPMENT OF LANGUAGE AND COORDINATION

AGE IN MONTHS	VOCALIZATION AND LANGUAGE	MOTOR DEVELOPMENT
4	Coos and chuckles.	Head self-supported; tonic neck reflex subsiding; can sit with pillow props on three sides.
6 to 9	Babbles; produces sounds such as "ma" or "da"; reduplication of sounds common.	Sits alone; pulls himself to standing; prompt unilateral reaching; first thumb opposition of grasp.
12 to 18	A small number of "words"; follows simple commands and responds to "no."	Stands momentarily alone; creeps; walks sideways when holding on to a railing; takes a few steps when held by hands; grasp, prehension, and release fully developed.
18 to 21	From about 20 words at 18 months to about 200 words at 21; points to many more objects; comprehends simple questions; forms two-word phrases.	Stance fully developed; gait stiff, propulsive, and precipitated; seats himself on child's chair with only fair aim, creeps downstairs backward; has difficulty building tower of three cubes; can throw a ball, but clumsily.

AGE IN MONTHS	VOCALIZATION AND LANGUAGE	MOTOR DEVELOPMENT
24 to 27	Vocabulary of 300 to 400 words; has two- to three-word phrases; uses prepositions and pronouns.	Runs but falls when making a sudden turn; can quickly alternate between stance, kneeling or sitting positions; walks stairs up and down, one foot forward only.
30 to 33	Fastest increase in vocabulary; three- to four-word sentences are common; word order, phrase structure, grammatical agreement approximate language of surroundings, but many utterances are unlike anything an adult would say.	Good hand and finger coordination; can move digits independently; manipulation of objects much improved; builds tower of six cubes.
36 to 39	Vocabulary of 1000 words or more; well-formed sentences using complex grammatical rules, although certain rules have not yet been fully mastered; grammatical mistakes are much less frequent; about 90 percent comprehensibility.	Runs smoothly with acceleration and deceleration; negotiates sharp and fast curves without difficulty; walks stairs by alternating feet; jumps 12 inches; can operate tricycle; stands on one foot for a few seconds.

SOURCE: From Eric Lenneberg, "The Natural History of Language," in F. Smith and G. Miller (eds.), *The Genesis of Language,* Cambridge, Mass.: MIT Press, 1966, Table 1, p. 222.

To analyze the effects of what we do to children we must consider the concepts of *heredity* and *environment*. The two are usually presented as opposites, but they are not as separate and contradictory as some theoretical discussions would indicate. In reality, heredity and environment are two sides of the same coin.

Take the example of the developing zygotes used at the start of this chapter. At first, all the cells are alike, but there is a genetic coding in each, which foretells many characteristics. This is the extreme case of heredity. But the actual differentiation of cells, which brings the genetic changes, comes about because of where each cell happens to be in the organism (its environment). In this case, the relationship between heredity and environment is more one of interaction than of opposition.

As another example, consider the baby duck, which instinctively follows its mother soon after birth. If some other object of the right size moves by at this time, the duckling will follow it and will never learn to follow the mother. If neither mother nor any other object passes by during the "critical period" for this learning, it never will learn to follow as normal ducks do.

Rats with identical genetic histories but raised in radically different environments often show behavioral differences. Environmental differences that persist through many generations favor certain naturally occurring mutations and thus alter the animals' genetic structure. Whole animals, just like individual cells, change in response to the environment. Change that takes place in one animal's lifetime is called *learning*, whereas change that requires adaptation over several generations is more likely to be called *genetic*. Both adaptations, however, are part of the biological scheme of evolution. Seen in this light, the distinction between innate behavior and learned behavior seems arbitrary (Alland, 1967). It may be more realistic to speak of three classes of behavior:

1. *Pure innate*. Such behavior remains the same generation after generation no matter what we do—for example, sexual behavior that serves to multiply a species.

2. *Innate-learned*. The ability to perform such behavior is also transmitted genetically, but the behavior appears only in response to environmental conditions. One might say that the envi-

ronment must "trigger" innate-learned behavior. Communication patterns, from bird songs to human language, fall into this category.

3. *Pure learned.* This type of behavior results from a single animal's successful adaptation to a set of conditions; it is not transmitted genetically. Ability to write, to read, and to speak eloquently seem to fall into this category.

Thus the child really has two kinds of biologically endowed abilities that help communicative development: (1) an innate capacity, which seems to be some form of knowledge about linguistic universals, and (2) strong general learning abilities relative to other animals. His learning strategies are important to mastering the pure-learned behavior associated with actual use of language.

The content of the child's environment, then, is important in two ways. First, his innate capacity to learn language behavior *must be triggered by the environment.* Just as the baby duck will not learn to follow without something to follow, the child will not learn to talk unless there are models around from which he can learn. Second, environment is all-important in regard to pure-learned behavior such as reading and writing. In this area, nothing is transmitted biologically, and each generation must learn anew.

Seen in this light, our roles as teachers and parents are vital. This view also makes it clearer what we must teach. There is no need to teach a child to talk; his biological heritage insures that he will grow up talking. Our job as teachers and parents is to teach children to talk effectively, in ways that benefit the individual and society alike.

RATIONALISTS VERSUS EMPIRICISTS

In recent years, a battle has raged between two schools of thought in child speech development. Empiricists, or behaviorists (e.g., Skinner, 1957), maintain that the mind is practically a blank slate at birth and that only experiences (stimuli) are important to the individual's behavior. Scholars in this camp hold that the child's environment is all-important in his learning to speak. They emphasize the role of the language the child hears and the responses of adults to the child's attempts to talk. Rationalists, or nativists (e.g., Chomsky, 1968), however, maintain that the individual's genetic structure determines that he will speak and that environmental variation is of little importance. Most of these scholars argue that the only environmental factor necessary for the child to learn to speak is exposure to some language. They regard such environmental factors as the mother's correction of the child's mistakes or her responses in general as relatively unimportant to his learning. This position may be summarized thus: While environmental factors can affect the quality of the language learned by the child, a "bad" environment cannot prevent the child from learning to speak if there is some language in the environment. Scholars in each camp expend much energy trying to discredit the other. This battling is unfortunate because the influences of heredity and environment are allies, not enemies. Both stimulate adaptive mechanisms, which help animals survive and prosper. Hopefully, future research will combine the strengths of both the rationalist and empiricist positions and give us a better picture of communication development.

SUMMARY

Several principles of developmental biology have application to speech development. The ability of children to make sentences grows much like the human organism. Man's communication system is remarkable, but many of its building blocks appear elsewhere in nature.

Still, man's speaking abilities are unique. No nonhumans talk; almost all humans do. The onset of language behavior in children is synchronized with motor development. Finally, all human languages share several basic aspects.

While human communication abilities are biological in nature and genetically transmitted, environment is important to speech development. Bad environments can harm even genetically determined behaviors. Further, even though children can learn to speak in almost any environment, only in supportive, teaching environments will they learn to read, write, or speak eloquently.

Read This

ALLAND, ALEXANDER. *Evolution and Human Behavior.* New York: Natural History Press, 1967.

Alland explains in readable language the principles of evolution and genetics and gives examples of the effects of these principles upon animal and human behavior.

LENNEBERG, ERIC. *Biological Foundations of Language.* New York: Wiley, 1967.

Lenneberg collects evidence from many areas of developmental biology to support the thesis that language behavior is species-specific to humans. His data range all the way from diagrams of the oral cavity to charts measuring brain growth to case histories of aphasic children.

MCNEILL, DAVID. "The Biological Background," *The Acquisition of Language.* New York: Harper & Row, 1970, chap. 4.

McNeill discusses human language in the context of other communication systems in nature, speculates about how man developed language, and evaluates attempts to make apes talk.

chapter 3

DEVELOPMENT OF THE SOUND SYSTEM

One of man's many language-connected abilities is to recognize that another person is speaking a foreign language. Indeed, we can often tell, just from the sound, what language it is. If you do not speak French or German, it is likely, nonetheless, that you recognize the sounds of these languages. A language's pattern of sounds is one of the things we must learn if we are to speak it. In this chapter, we shall explore the process of children's acquisition of the sounds of the language. We consider first what the child has to learn, and second, what happens in the learning process.

PHONEMES

Every language is made up of a limited number of sounds—the building blocks of language. They can be put together in various combinations to make up the words of the language. Approximately 43 sounds make up all the words used in English. Other languages have different numbers of sounds—Spanish, for example, uses about 24. Some languages share sounds—for example, English and Spanish both use the sound we represent by the letter *p*. However, other sounds are different. Many Spanish speakers have difficulty hearing the difference between the vowel sounds in the English words *leave* and *live* because these are not separate sounds in Spanish. The sounds used to make words are called *phonemes*. Phonemes, which are shared by all the speakers of a given language, vary among languages. English and Spanish sound different because they are made up partly of different sets of phonemes.

PLACE AND MANNER OF ARTICULATION

There are many ways to describe language sounds. A physicist might describe sounds in terms of pure acoustical properties. In analyzing phonemes, however, it is easiest to classify sounds according to where and how they are articulated. Make the sound /p/. Notice that the sound happens when you bring your lips together and release a puff of air. Thus, the *place of articulation* is the lips; the *manner of articulation* is to stop air and then release it.

Table 2 classifies the consonants of English according to place and manner of articulation. At the top of the table, sounds are classified according to *place* of articulation. *Bilabial* sounds are made with the lips (e.g., / p / and / b /). *Labiodental* sounds are made by contact between the lower lip and upper teeth (e.g., /f/ and / v /). Many sounds are made by contact between the tongue and some part of the mouth. *Dental* sounds are made with tongue and teeth (e.g., / th /, as in "think"); *alveolar* sounds are made with tongue and alveolar ridge (behind the top teeth; e.g., / t / and / d /). *Palatal* sounds are made by raising the tongue toward the palate, or roof of the mouth. The initial sound in words such as "yes" and "yellow" is a palatal sound. Behind the palate is the velum, or soft palate. Sounds made by contact between the back of the tongue and the velum (e.g., / k / and / g /) are called *velar*. Even further down the throat than the velum are the vocal cords. *Glottal* sounds are made only with the vocal cords (e.g., the initial sound in "happy" and "how").

The terms in the left-hand column of Table 2 refer to the manner in which a sound is made. *Stop* sounds, for example, are made by closing off the flow of air completely, then releasing it. As you can see by looking across the table, stop sounds can be made at many locations in the mouth. *Fricative* sounds are made by narrowing the opening of the mouth so that the flow of air is not entirely blocked, but is obstructed. Fricatives produce a "hissing" noise due to the turbulence of the air passing through the

table **2**
PLACE AND MANNER OF ARTICULATION
IN ENGLISH CONSONANTS

	BILABIAL	LABIO-DENTAL	DENTAL	ALVEOLAR	PALATAL	VELAR	GLOTTAL
STOP	p b			t d		k g	
FRICATIVE		f v	th	s z	sh zh		h
AFFRICATE				ch j			
GLIDE	w wh				y		
LIQUID				l	r		
NASAL	m			n		ng	

small opening. Consonant sounds that combine the properties of stops and fricatives are called *affricates*. Affricates are made by cutting off the air flow completely, as in a stop, then releasing it through a very small opening, as in a fricative. Affricates are accompanied by the hissing sound typical of fricatives, as can be heard by pronouncing "church" and "judge." Sounds made by closing the mouth at some point and allowing air to escape through the nose are called *nasals*. Nasals are classified according to where the closure in the mouth occurs. Some consonants are much like vowels in that no closure occurs in the mouth. These

are the *liquids* (e.g., / l / and / r /) and the *glides* (e.g., / w /,
/ wh /, and / y /). Glides are so much like vowels that they are
often called *semivowels*.

Consonant sounds are classified according to place and manner
of articulation; vowel sounds are classified according to the
height of the tongue in the mouth (high, mid, low) and whether
the highest point of the tongue is nearer the front or the back of
the mouth. One main difference between consonants and vowels
is that for vowels there is never a closure in the mouth, while
there often is for consonants. Vowel classification is often represented by the vowel diagram (see Table 3). In this diagram, the
vowels are classified as high, mid, low, and front vs. back. For example, / i / as in "beat" is a high front vowel, while / a / as in
"hot" is a low back vowel.

table 3
ENGLISH VOWELS

	FRONT	CENTRAL	BACK
HIGH	/i/as in "beat"		/u/as in "boo"
	/ɪ/as in "bit"		/ʊ/as in "good"
MID	/e/as in "bait"	/ʌ/ as in "much" /ə/ as in "*a*rrest"	/o/as in "boat"
	/ɛ/as in "bet"		/ɔ/as in "ball"
LOW	/æ/ as in "bat"		/a/ as in "father"

DISTINCTIVE FEATURES

Suppose you decide to describe the sound / p / in Table 2. You could say several things about the sound. First, the sound is a consonant, not a vowel. Second, it is articulated by bringing the lips together (bilabial). Third, it is articulated as a "stop." To summarize, / p / is a *consonant* and a *bilabial stop*.

The sound / b / also has all of these features but is different from / p / in *voicing*. If the vocal cords vibrate when a sound is made, the sound is voiced. If you put your fingers lightly over your throat—where the Adam's apple is—and make the sounds / p / and / b /, you should feel the vocal cords vibrate on / b /. The sound / b / is voiced; / p / is not.

We could describe the sounds / b / and / p / in terms of all the features we have discussed. The description might resemble Table 4. Looking at sounds according to articulatory features is called *distinctive feature analysis*. Distinctive features provide an economical way to describe sounds. Table 4, for example, tells us that the only difference between / p / and / b / is the voicing feature. Otherwise, the two sounds are alike.

table 4
DISTINCTIVE FEATURE ANALYSIS

	p	b
CONSONANT	+	+
VOWEL	−	−
LABIAL	+	+
STOP	+	+
VOICING	−	+

Not all articulatory features will be distinctive in a given language. For example, / t / can be made with the tongue against the alveolar ridge or with the tongue against the teeth (if the tongue touches the teeth, / t / is said to be dentalized). You can make / t / with the lips rounded or not rounded. You can also make / t / *aspirated* or *unaspirated*. An aspirated sound is one that is accompanied by a puff of air. You can feel this if you hold your hand about an inch away from your lips and pronounce "toy." Now, with your hand still there, pronounce "stop." The / t / in "toy" is aspirated; in "stop" it is not. All of these features of articulation can vary, and yet the sound produced will still be recognized by speakers of English as / t /. We do not make any distinction between aspirated / t / and unaspirated / t /, but in some Arabic languages they are regarded as different sounds, just as / t / and / d / are regarded as different sounds in English. The point here is that in every language some sound differences are *distinctive,* while other differences will be nondistinctive. As mentioned above, aspiration is nondistinctive for English speakers. We do not have two words that are different because one has an aspirated / t / and one has an unaspirated / t /. However, other sound features are distinctive for English speakers. For example, as noted previously, *voicing* is a distinctive feature in English, but there are languages in which voicing is not a distinctive feature, and to speakers of these languages, "beat" and "peat" might sound like the same word.

Many other sound features are distinctive sounds for speakers of English. An oversimplified view of the theory has been presented here. For more information, see Jakobson and Halle (1956) or Chomsky and Halle (1968).

SOUND ACQUISITION

The child seems to learn the phoneme system of his language through discovering distinctive features, which is a process of *differentiation.*

Phoneme differentiation does not begin until sounds are used meaningfully—in words. The first distinction the child makes is usually between vowel and consonant. One example of this, which appears early in children's speech, is the distinction between /p/ as in *p*it and /a/ as in *f*ather. Using this distinction, the child can say "pa" or "papa." Once begun, the process of differentiation proceeds rapidly. The next distinction made may be

between nasal and nonnasal consonants—in the form of distin-guishing / p / from / m /.

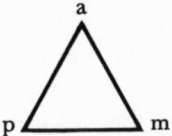

Now the phonemes / pa / and / ma / —and usually the words des-ignating the child's parents: "papa" and "mama"—are available for use. Both / p / and / m / are made with the lips, so the child soon makes a labial–nonlabial distinction in the form of using / f / or / s / in contrast with / p / and / m /. Whatever the sounds he first uses (they may vary from the examples given here), the child can make three or four sounds, and his "first words" can mean a variety of things. Valued objects such as baby bottles or cookies may be named "ba" or "sa" or some other easy-to-say form.

The child does not make any vowel contrasts until he has mas-tered several consonants. The first vowel distinction is likely to be between *wide-open mouth* (e.g., / a /) and *narrow-opening* (e.g., / i /).

Jakobson (1956) says that these first few contrasts are language universals (in the sense discussed in Chapter 2). Some support for this view is found in the fact that many languages use words sim-ilar to "mama" and "papa" to refer to parents.

More important than particular sounds is the idea that the dif-ferentiation process for learning these sounds may be universal—may spring from general rules of sound which describe all languages. In other words, all languages have the basic kinds of sound contrasts discussed for English: between stops and nasals and fricatives for consonants; between wide and narrow for vowels. This universality explains why children make these distinctions first.

This does not mean that all languages have the same phonemes, nor does it mean that all children learn each contrast at the same age. Children vary in *rate* of acquisition, but *order* of learning of certain contrasts seems to be the same. As the child develops more sound contrasts, he progresses further into a specific language such as English or French and further away from the early universal contrasts. The sound contrasts could be arranged hierarchically, with very broad, universal contrasts, such as vowel vs. consonant occurring first, and very fine, more language-specific contrasts, such as voiced vs. unvoiced sounds, occurring later. Jakobson's theory explains the acquisition of the broad, early contrasts, but for a treatment of later acquisition we must look elsewhere.

Distinctive feature analysis alone is not enough to specify all that the child must learn about the sounds of his language. As we mentioned earlier, not all the articulatory features of sounds are distinctive for any given language. Features that are not distinctive—that do not serve to contrast different words in the language—are specified by linquistic rules. For example, aspiration is not a distinctive feature for speakers of English. A general phonological rule of English states that all initial voiceless stops are aspirated—that is, in words such as "tin" and "pin," the first sounds will be aspirated. There are no contrasting words that begin with unaspirated / t / or / p /. When the child learns to say "tin," he must learn that / t / is voiceless (to distinguish it from "din"), and he must learn that it is an alveolar stop rather than a fricative (to distinguish it from "sin"). However, he need not learn that in this particular word / t / is aspirated, because initial / t / is always aspirated in English. Once the child has mastered the general rule, he does not have to be concerned about every particular instance of the sound. Another rule of English is that stop sounds are always unaspirated after / s /. A child learning to say "stop" or "spat" need not learn for each individual word that the sound coming after / s / is unaspirated. It will always be so. All he must learn is the rule. There are no contrasts between words beginning / s / -aspirated stop vs.

/s/-unaspirated stop, so the child does not learn this through a series of contrasts, as he learns distinctive features. He must, instead, somehow acquire knowledge of the system of rules that governs how we put sounds together to make words in English. We have given only a hint of what some of these rules are like. We know very little about how the child learns these rules and the order in which they are acquired. However, it is clear that if the child is going to speak English, he must abide by them.

EARLY WORD FORMATION

As most parents can tell you, children often have difficulty with the sounds of the language when they are first learning to make words. The whole idea of "baby talk" is based on this fact, so when the mother says "Bwing Mommy the wabbit," she may be imitating the mistakes made by the child. Some children quickly overcome these early difficulties, but others may continue to have trouble with certain sounds even after they have started school.

The kinds of mistakes children make in their early words can be described systematically. According to Franke (1912), children's first words are one-consonant forms. The consonants / m /, / b /, and / p / are among the first to appear and they are used in consonant-vowel or consonant-vowel-consonant forms. Although children in the first stages of word formation may be able to articulate as many as eight consonants properly, they will never use more than one in any individual word. It is as if the child cannot change place or manner of articulation within words. This phenomenon can be seen clearly in one of Franke's examples of children's pronunciation of the German word "baum" (tree). Of three children observed, one said "mamau," one said "bau," and one said "maum." Although each of the three is different, they have in common the fact that a word with two consonants was changed to a one-consonant form by dropping one consonant or substituting for it.

The rules for sound omission or substitution in early word formation reflect this one-consonant tendency. When a word the child is trying to say has more than one consonant, he eliminates all consonants except one. Sometimes he substitutes this one for the others. Thus the English word "cup" becomes "pup" or "cuc." Several factors influence which consonant in a word will be retained. Generally, the consonant most likely to be retained is the middle one (the / n / in "pencil," for example), followed by the first, then the last. Another factor influencing consonant retention is difficulty of articulation. Consonants that are hard for children to make (e.g., / r /) will be dropped or substituted for in children's early speech. Finally, in a word with many syllables, only stressed syllables are likely to be retained. Thus, "elephant" may become "ef," or "telephone" may become "te" or "fo."

The distortions little children produce when they try to say some words are not simply a result of the fact that some sounds are too hard for them to make. By the age of two, many children are able to articulate clearly all the sounds of the language. However, there is more to making words than this. Putting sounds together is not the same as saying sounds in isolation, and children must learn which sounds to use and how to put them together before it can be said that they have learned the sound system of a language. This suggests that the process of babbling, which used to be considered essential to speech development, does not insure that the child will be able to articulate clearly when he begins to make words. When the infant lies in his crib making sounds to himself, he may make a large range of sounds, even the / r / and / l / sounds, which are quite difficult for many four-year-olds. But the fact that a baby can make a sound in isolation as he babbles does not insure that he will be able to use the sound in combination with other sounds to make words. Deaf children babble for several months, just as hearing children do, yet the deaf child will not develop spoken language as a young child unless he can be helped to hear it. Babbling just seems to be one of those cute characteristics of babyhood—fun for parents and probably fun for baby, too, but not sufficient to insure good articulation in later stages.

SUMMARY

Children must learn about sounds before they make words because sounds are the building blocks of a language. The sound unit of a language is called a *phoneme*. There are several ways to describe phonemes, among them classification by place and manner of articulation and distinctive feature analysis.

Children seem to acquire the sound system through learning a system of contrasts, beginning with the major contrast between consonants and vowels and proceeding through finer and finer contrasts until they have learned to contrast the distinctive features of the language they are learning. This learning by differentiation is accompanied by the acquisition of the rules that govern the use of nondistinctive sound features.

When they are learning to talk, children often distort the sounds of words. Such distortion is attributable to several factors, among them that children appear to have difficulty changing the place or manner of articulation of consonants within a word, and that some sounds are simply harder for children to articulate than others.

Read This

JAKOBSON, ROMAN, and MORRIS HALLE. *Fundamentals of Language.* The Hague: Mouton, 1956.

In the section on phonology and phonetics, Jakobson and Halle extend and elaborate the distinctive feature approach to children's learning of phonology.

LEWIS, M. M. *Language, Thought and Personality in Infancy and Childhood.* New York: Basic Books, 1963.

Lewis provides an excellent and readable account of sounds made by children—largely based upon observation of his own children.

chapter 4

DEVELOPMENT OF SYNTAX:
WHAT REALLY HAPPENED BEHIND
THE TRANSFORMATIONAL TREE?

The growth of children's speech can be described in terms of the structure, or syntax, of the sentence spoken. Recent research in syntactic development has produced dramatic insights into child speech. For this, we are heavily indebted to linguist Noam Chomsky, whose theories have created new emphases in several areas of thought about sentence structure. This chapter discusses a few highlights of this approach and describes how these concepts have been applied to the child's development of grammar.

SYNTAX

Each of us knows a great deal about sentence structure. You may protest: "I don't know a thing about sentence structure—I can't even diagram complex sentences!" Yet you demonstrate your knowledge of syntax dozens of times each day.

To show yourself how much you know, answer this question: Which of these sentences looks wrong to you?

1. The child aggravates his mother.
2. The aggravates child his mother.

Sentence 2 is obviously the wrong one. Because the words are out of order, it makes little sense. You noticed this right away, even though you may not be able to explain why. This is because you have *grammatical intuition,* which means that you know about the structures of sentences *even though you do not know what you know about it.* You know it implicitly. We can tell that you know the rules of syntax because you obey them every time you speak. You never say sentences such as 2. This shows that you know such sentences are not grammatical in structure. Your grammatical intuition is so trustworthy that linguists' most common analysis procedure is to ask nonlinguists (you) to evaluate intuitively the structures of sentences. For example, you might be asked what you notice about these two sentences:

3. Americans love anarchy.
4. Anarchy is loved by Americans.

You probably notice two things. First, the two sentences say the same thing. Second, they are different in structure. If we gave you the sentence

5. Walruses swallow ice.

which has the same structure as 3, "Americans love anarchy," and asked you to produce the structural equivalent of 4, you would have little trouble supplying the answer:

6. Ice is swallowed by walruses.

which means that you understand intuitively the structural relationships between these sentences. You have that understanding even though you may never have heard of a *passive transformation,* which is the linguistic name for the operation you just performed.

The body of intuitive knowledge about grammar that each of us possesses is called *linguistic competence.* All speakers possess competence in their language, although competence is never seen. Suppose we gave you sentences 1 and 2 above and asked you which was wrong—but you had failed to answer. We could *not* say you did not know that part of grammar. We could only say you did not answer the question. *Maybe* your competence is deficient, but more likely you just did not answer for some other reason: You are angry at us for being boring writers, you forgot the question, you'd feel weird answering a question asked in a book, or something like that. All these are problems of *lin-*

guistic performance. The problem is not a lack of knowledge on your part, but simply the failure to show what you know.

This is an important issue in studying children, who can be very uncooperative about demonstrating their competence. In one study, an experimenter asked a child of about age two, "Which is right, 'two shoes' or 'two shoe'?" The child responded enthusiastically, "Pop goes the weasel!" (Brown and Bellugi, 1964). Every child language researcher has lived through hundreds of similarly exasperating moments. How can you say that the child in the "two shoes" example did not know correct plural form? Obviously you cannot. Much of child language research consists of trying to trick children into showing what they know.

Which leads us to one of the central questions of syntax: _What is it that we know when we know the structure of a sentence?_

DEEP STRUCTURE AND SURFACE STRUCTURE

Every sentence actually has two levels of structure, or syntax. The sentence you see going from one word to the next across a page is the _surface structure_ level. But sentences also have an underlying level called _deep structure_. When a child or adult knows the structure of a sentence, he understands both levels.

To demonstrate that sentences really have two levels of structure, examine these:

7. The elf swung the hammer.
8. The hammer was swung by the elf.

Obviously, these two sentences look different—they have different surface structures. Yet they also mean the same thing—both refer to the same organism grasping the same tool in the same appendage and performing the same action. So in the underlying level (deep structure), these two sentences are the same. Two sentences that are different on the surface yet mean the same thing must have two levels of structure.

The same trick works the other way. Take this well-known sentence,

9. The shooting of the hunters was terrible.

This sentence has only one surface structure, but two plausible meanings: (a) hunters were shooting inaccurately, (b) hunters were being shot (to the dismay of onlookers). Each of these meanings corresponds to a different underlying structure. In this case, there are two deep structures, one surface structure.

You know (intuitively) that there are two levels of sentence structure, or you would not have understood these examples.

As he grows, a child needs to understand sentence syntax on both deep and surface structure levels. Any theoretical account of his communication development must explain how he manages to acquire such understanding. This is a problem because we do not know precisely what deep structure is like. We do know that one way to describe the structure of any single sentence is to divide it into its constituent parts—structure is by definition the relationship between parts. Take, for example, this sentence:

10. The linguist described a sentence.

If we asked you what would be the most natural way to divide this sentence into two parts, you would probably divide it as follows:

The linguist   described a sentence.

These two parts are the main structural constituents of the sentence. The first part is a noun phrase (subject), and the second part is a verb phrase (predicate). If we wanted to analyze this sentence further, we might take the verb and divide it:

described   a sentence

We could continue such subdividing until we ran out of words. You could intuitively tell where to divide each part of the sentence. These dividing places indicate aspects of its syntax.

This kind of analysis helps us to understand the structure of this one sentence. But to understand what the child is learning about sentence structure in general, we need to be able to describe much more than one sentence. We need to describe the entire set of possibilities in the language. We can attempt this more powerful description by making educated guesses (hypotheses) about the structures used in English sentences. Such hypotheses are called *rules of syntax,* or phrase structure rules.

It must be emphasized that these are not prescriptive rules. Unlike highway speed limits or rules for agreement of verb tense that you learned in high-school English, linguistic rules do not tell us what we should do. Rather, they describe, like the "rule" that you rarely talk on elevators and that you face the person you are speaking to. Linguistic rules are not rules because lawmakers or schoolteachers say they are, but because they provide an accurate description of the actual structures in human sentences.

HOW PHRASE STRUCTURE RULES WORK

Phrase structure rules divide sentences or phrases into two parts, just as we did with sentence 10. But phrase structure rules are more general and abstract. For example, instead of dividing sentence 10 as we did, we could write the following rule:

(a) SENTENCE → NOUN PHRASE + VERB PHRASE

The arrow → is a lot like an equals sign. It shows that the item on the left (SENTENCE) can be rewritten, or represented, as the two items on the right. In the case of our sample sentence, the NOUN PHRASE is "The linguist" and the VERB PHRASE is "described a sentence."

We can continue to divide this sample sentence as we did before, using this rule:

(b) VERB PHRASE → VERB + NOUN PHRASE
          (described)   (a sentence)

Note that the two groups of words left unanalyzed in this sample sentence ("the linguist" and "a sentence") are both noun phrases identical in structure. We can describe these phrases as follows:

(c) NOUN PHRASE → ARTICLE + NOUN
          (the, a)   (linguist, sentence)

At this point we have provided a set of rules that describes not only this sentence but also many others of the same structure. For example, these same three rules could apply to "The boy hit the ball," "The walrus suffered a stroke," or "A giraffe is an animal." By adding just a few more rules to this set, we could describe many of the most common sentences spoken in the English language.

We have gone through this exercise to illustrate that a small number of rules form the basis of what we know about syntax. In order to understand sentence structure, children have to know these rules. How children develop knowledge of these syntax rules is the subject of most of this chapter.

Before we get to that, however, we need to add one qualification. You recall that sentences have two levels of structure, deep structure and surface structure. Phrase structure rules describe only deep structure. So if we are analyzing sentences such as:

11. Teachers hit students.
12. Students are hit by teachers.

(which have the same deep structure) they both would be described using the same phrase structure rules. To talk about the ways these sentences are different from each other (they are different in surface structure only), we must discuss a different kind of rule, called a *transformation*.

TRANSFORMATIONS

The differences between sentences 11 and 12 are that in 12 the subject and object ("students" and "teachers") have switched places with each other, and the words "are" and "by" surround the verb ("hit"). All these operations can be shown in one rule, called a *passive transformation*, which can be condensed to look like this:

noun #1 + verb + noun #2 → noun #2 + are + verb + by + noun #1

This may look complex (tricky) on paper, but you did it easily on page 35. Here is another example of how a transformation works. Deep structures are like a stack of propositions that express the sentence meanings. If you say the phrase:

13. the big red dirty truck

the deep structure of the phrase would contain something like:

    i. the truck is big.
   ii. the truck is red.
  iii. the truck is dirty.

Obviously it would be cumbersome if we had to say all that. So we use the *adjective transformation,* which deletes all the words that we would have to use over and over, and places the adjective in front of the noun it modifies.

There are many kinds of transformations. Most sentences employ several of them. They greatly aid the economy of spoken language. Transformations are also the key to understanding the relationships between affirmative sentences ("I like you"), negative sentences ("I do not like you"), and questions ("Do I like you?"). Because asking questions and saying no are both important to children, how they learn these transformations is important.

To summarize: We can describe the structure of the English language using phrase structure rules and transformations. We can use these same rules to describe what the child is learning when he learns syntax. We are now sufficiently armed with jargon to face that problem—which is, after all, the purpose of this chapter.

CHILDREN'S SYNTAX

When the child first begins speaking words, his utterances are generally one word long: "Daddy," "bye-bye," "cookie." This has been explained by saying that these words are simply imitations of things adults have said. There is some truth to this point of view, especially with the child's first half dozen words. We are all familiar with the scene in which the child, playing alone, says "mama-mama." The mother, overhearing, leaps to her feet and hugs the confused child profusely for his "first word." This kind of reinforcement is undoubtedly responsible for some words.

However, this view seems to imply that first words (which are almost all nouns) are simple "labels"—conditioned connections to the objects named. Most linguists reject this idea, saying that first words are really little sentences, or *holophrases.*

In this view, a child at the stage of *holophrastic speech* is saying immature sentences, which make statements, in addition to giving labels. When the child says "cookie," he is not simply labeling, but stating a desire. He is more likely to be satisfied if we give him the cookie than if we respond "Right! It's a cookie."

The point is that a child at this age, although he may only say single words, uses these words as sentences. And the single-word sentence, plus the context in which it is said, usually provides enough information so that we can understand what the child is saying.

Looking at single-word utterances as little sentences is interesting in light of the discussion of biology in Chapter 3. The holophrase is a lot like the single-celled zygote. The zygote is the common undifferentiated beginning of a human life. The holophrase is the common undifferentiated beginning of the structure of human language. Within the zygote is a genetic code that will determine the growth of the organism. If a holophrase is an entire sentence, then it too contains implicitly the coded structure of the entire language.

This analogy is supported by the fact that most single-word utterances are nouns. Nouns, as McNeill (1970, p. 25) points out, are the only kind of word that can be used in every structural position of a sentence. Nouns can be used as subjects ("The toy is mine"), objects ("I want the toy"), or modifiers ("The toy box is full"). No other part of speech can do this. Growing organisms start out with only one kind of cell. Human language starts out with only one structural category of words. The next step, both for cell and sentence, is differentiation.

Pivot Structures *

The process of differentiation, discussed earlier in connection with phonological development, can be seen in syntactic development when the single structural class of holophrastic speech is differentiated into more specialized syntactic classes. In this

* The information in this section is mostly from McNeill (1966, 1970). Any inaccuracies, of course, belong to us.

scheme of structural differentiation, the central syntactic class of words is called the *pivot* class. The pivot class reveals itself when the child starts to speak two-word sentences. Here are a few that might be typical:

> My ball.
> Read book.
> Here truck.

Note that all the second words in these utterances are nouns. In one-word speech, you will recall, most items were nouns, and the few that were not nouns were a mixed bag of every other grammatical category. When the child talks as in the three examples above, he has made a differentiation between the nouns and everything else. He now has two grammatical classes: nouns, called the *open class*, and the mixed bag of leftovers, called the *pivot class*.

A rule of syntax describing the three utterances above would be written this way:

S	$\rightarrow$	P	+	O
(sentence)	(is rewritten as)	(pivot word)		(open-class word)

It should be pointed out that a child of this age (about eighteen months) also produces little sentences which are two nouns, or open-class words—for example, "Mommy sock."

$$S \rightarrow O + O$$

There are also some sentences in which the open word is first: "Candy mine."

$$S \rightarrow O + P$$

But *never,* and this is largely the power of this scheme, does the child say a pivot word by itself or with other pivot words. Note that this argument is slightly circular: If a pivot word appeared with another P word we probably would say that one of them must be an O word. Science advances by small steps.

Let us summarize: By constructing this little two-class grammar to describe the speech of an eighteen-month-old child, we can see that he has differentiated holophrases into two categories of words, pivot and open classes. It should be mentioned here that the concept of a two-class grammar has been challenged, perhaps most effectively by Lois Bloom (1971). Her primary objection to this view of the child's speech is that it is based on a distributional analysis—that is, it is a description based simply on which words are used together (how they are distributed in sentences) and ignores the question of how the child is *using* the words. This viewpoint will be treated more completely in Chapter 5. However, it should be pointed out that although a distributional analysis may provide an oversimplified view of the child's speech, the observation that distributional categories exist is not denied in Bloom's criticism.

The next step in development is further differentiation of the mixed-bag pivot class. The open class stays quite stable. About three months after pivot speech begins, the child has differentiated the pivot class into three classes—articles (a, the), some demonstrative pronouns (this, that), and a further mixed bag of leftovers, which can be called Pivot 2. Three more months and Pivot 2 class has itself been differentiated into three more classes: adjectives (big, red), possessive pronouns (my, mine, your), and a mixed bunch called Pivot 3. Figure 1 (adapted from McNeill, 1970) traces the differentiation of grammatical classes during the second year of the child's life.

One more extension of the analogy between the biological development of life and the grammatical development of the sentence is appropriate here. The genetic code in the zygote predetermines the properties of the growing animal; thus each differentiation that takes place is appropriate to what the final product will be. Similarly, each differentiation made as the child's syntax develops is consistent and appropriate to set up distinctions that will be made later—leading to adult sentence structure. All these factors indicate that language develops in a predetermined manner, essentially controlled by our genetic structure.

For more detailed descriptions of child syntax, see Brown, Cazden, and Bellugi (1969) and McNeill (1970).

Learning Transformations

In the discussion of *linguistic universals* (Chapter 2), it was noted that all languages are alike in many ways even though they are not mutually understandable. It happens that the parts of syntax that are universals (relationship of subject and predicate, that verb phrases contain verbs and noun phrases, etc.) are nearly all aspects of *deep structure*.

Because surface structure is made up of deep structure plus transformations, it is theoretically attractive to say that deep structures unfold in child speech at a very early age (and that their development is genetically determined) whereas transformations are mastered later (and are more a result of learning). Evidence suggests that this does happen.

When transformations do develop, however, they unfold in a predetermined, rule-governed manner much like the unfolding of

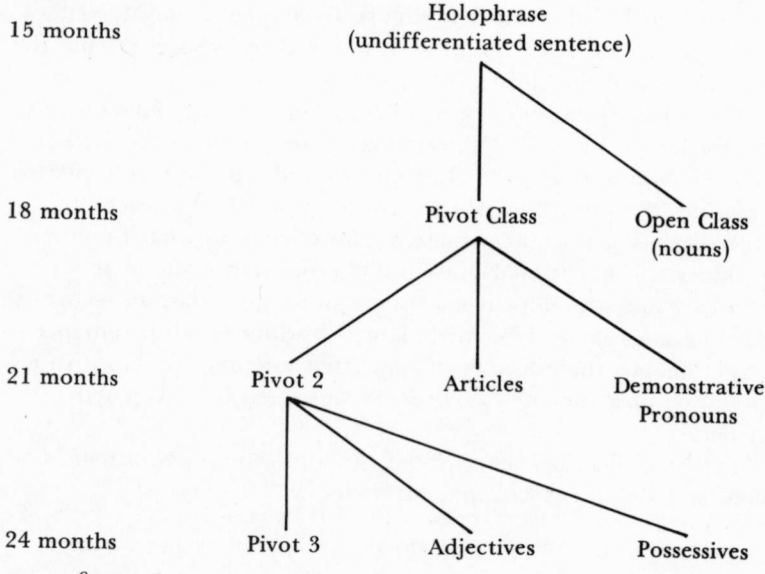

CHILD'S
APPROXIMATE
AGE

15 months — Holophrase (undifferentiated sentence)

18 months — Pivot Class — Open Class (nouns)

21 months — Pivot 2 — Articles — Demonstrative Pronouns

24 months — Pivot 3 — Adjectives — Possessives

figure 1
DIFFERENTIATION OF CLASSES IN CHILD SYNTAX

earlier structures. The transformations that have been most carefully studied are questions and negation. Both develop through
three stages (Klima and Bellugi, 1966). In the first stage, the
function is performed and the meaning gets across, but the structure is very rudimentary and simple. Questions are accomplished
by rising intonation at the end of a sentence:

> Doggie gone?
> Taste it?

Negation is accomplished by simply putting the word *no* in front
of the declarative sentence.

> No night night. (Brian's favorite)
> No go outside.

During the second stage, children begin to put some of the verbal machinery into place, but they make many quaint "mistakes"
in use of pronouns and auxiliary verbs.

> Why me go?
> Who milk is dat?
> Do like grapefruit?
> That not red.
> I no want envelope.

In the third stage, most of the necessary auxiliary verbs and
pronouns are present in adult form, although they sometimes
disagree in number and appear out of adult order.

> Who took them all down?
> Did you drink your coffee?
> How can he be a doctor?
> I am not a doctor.
> This not ice cream.
> You don't want some supper.

Surprisingly, for all children studied, these stages have been
mastered in the same order. This suggests that children must
have some basically universal learning strategies that they bring
to bear on mastering syntax. When we examine some of these
learning strategies closely, we begin to see some of the linguistic
"mistakes" discussed above in a new light.

Strategies for Learning Syntax

Children's speech "mistakes" can give us insights into their style of learning. One of Brian's first words was "bow-wow," referring to four-legged barking creatures. Shortly after he began to use this word, he started applying it in reference to all four-legged furry creatures: horses, cats, everything. It was as if he had just discovered the class "four-legged creatures" and decided to call it "bow-wow." Adult response to his generalization was, of course, mixed, ranging from "That's right, that's a bow-wow," to "No, that's a cow." Through this feedback process, Brian was forced to differentiate among varieties of animals, only one of which was "bow-wow." After three months of interesting variations on this theme, Brian could successfully name several classes of animals.

Brian's problem was that he had a good idea, but he overgeneralized its application. An overgeneralization sequence much like this one occurs in many aspects of language development and explains many child errors in speaking. Children use "strong verbs" (frequently occurring irregular verbs such as *to run*) correctly when they first learn to talk. But later, after they learn regular verbs, children overgeneralize the rules of past tense (for example) from the regular to irregular verbs: "I runned."

Slobin (1966) observed similar overgeneralization sequences occurring in the language-learning strategies of Russian children:

> Overregularizations are rampant in the child's learning of Russian morphology. . . . For example, not only must the child learn an instrumental case ending for each masculine, feminine and neuter singular and plural noun and adjective, but within each of these subcategories there are several different phonologically conditioned suffixes. The child's solution is to seize upon one suffix at first—probably the most frequent and / or most clearly marked acoustically—and use it for every instance of that particular grammatical category. (pp. 137–138)

Slobin uses the term "inflectional imperialism" to refer to this tendency for one affix to drive others temporarily out of usage. What is really happening is simple. The child formulates a rule, finds cases in which it works well, and immediately generalizes its use to many situations—in some of which it is inappropriate. This process is much like what social scientists do in the "implications" section of a research report. In overgeneralizing rules of grammar, the child is in error only in the same sense that thirty-year-old journal articles sometimes seem naïve. Still, modern theories spring directly from the scientific insights of thirty years ago, and adult language springs from the overgeneralized hypotheses of children.

A final note: Overgeneralization, as discussed here, is the flip side of differentiation. It is only through rule-inducing overgeneralization that the child can produce grammatical categories sufficiently broad or inclusive enough to divide. Each differentiation creates new categories to be overgeneralized. Each of these concepts is meaningful only in terms of the other—like yin and yang, East and West. The cycle of overgeneralization–differentiation is natural and self-perpetuating. In development of grammar, each repetition of the cycle generates information that is more specific, detailed, reality-centered, and useful.

Later Acquisition of Syntax

By age four or five, at the latest, the child has acquired *most* of the basic principles of syntax. Recent studies (C. Chomsky, 1969; Kessel, 1969) have demonstrated, however, that the child does not master some syntactic rules until as late as age ten or twelve. Syntax acquisition in later years is less rapid and dramatic than in early stages of development. Finishing the job of acquiring the grammar seems more like learning to read or to multiply than it seems like early syntactic development. It appears to be more a process of individual learning.

From our speculations about overgeneralization learning strategies, we could predict the principles of syntax that are learned late. They are not rules of far-reaching application, but rather specific *exceptions* to such rules, which are important in only a few special instances. For example, sentences using the word *promise*

Bozo promises Donald to do a somersault.

are exceptional in syntax. Such sentences are an exception to a general rule called the *minimal distance principle,* which can be illustrated by this sentence:

Bozo tells Donald to do a somersault.

In this sentence, the subject of the second verb ("do") is the noun *closest* to it ("Donald"). This means simply that Donald is going to do the somersault. In the "promise" sentence (the exception), it is *Bozo* who is going to tumble. Because the "promise" sentence is exceptional, children learn how to handle it later than the "tell" sentence.

The child learns these specific exceptions to syntax rules late —often in school. And the way he learns them seems radically different from early syntax acquisition. This difference is discussed further in Chapter 8.

COMPREHENSION AND PRODUCTION

There are basically two ways to find out what a child knows about grammar. You can tell him to do something, and if he does it, you know he understands (comprehends) what you said. However, production tasks consist of trying to find ways to get children to use language spontaneously, to show what they know. Both techniques are widely used, and data resulting from both techniques have been lumped together in this chapter. For instance, most data on pivot structures in development come from sentences children said spontaneously. The data on late development are mostly comprehension based.

This distinction deserves mention because if you tested the same child for both comprehension and production, he would probably understand more than he could say, just as when we read we understand words that we never say ourselves. This fact often makes it difficult to form conclusions about when specific rules are mastered. Additional research may correct this problem.

✳SUMMARY✳

Linguists distinguish between competence (abilities underlying language behavior) and performance (the actual observable act of speaking). When a speaker knows the syntax of a language, he actually knows two levels of structure—surface structure and deep structure. The syntax of sentences is best described by rules.

Phrase structure rules describe deep structure, and transformational rules describe the operations performed upon deep structures to obtain surface structures.

Children begin speaking by uttering single words. Calling these words holophrases indicates the supposition that these words are implicitly sentences—that the word and contextual cues add up to full-sentence meanings.

The child's next step in syntax development is to differentiate the holophrase class of words into open-class words (nouns) and pivot-class words (everything else). Following this, the pivot class itself is further differentiated. About six months after the beginning of pivot speech, the child has evolved word classes out of the pivot class. This entire process is reminiscent of the evolution of a human life from a single cell through differentiation. The child's major learning strategy in syntactic development is an overgeneralization process complementary to this differentiation.

Later syntax acquisition, although less rapid and dramatic, is tied more to learning individual instances than are early acquisition processes. The items learned late are ordinarily exceptions to syntactic rules.

Read This

BROWN, ROGER. *Psycholinguistics*. New York: Free Press, 1970.
   The first half of this book is a collection of some of the most important scholarly papers on syntax acquisition.
CHOMSKY, NOAM. *Language and Mind*. New York: Harcourt Brace Jovanovich, 1968.
   This book, a printed version of three lectures on the history of linguistics, is Chomsky's most readable introduction to his theory of syntax. Available in paperback. An even briefer introduction appears in a magazine article with the same title in *Psychology Today* (February 1968).
MCNEILL, DAVID. "Developmental Psycholinguistics," in Frank Smith and George Miller (eds.), *The Genesis of Language*. Cambridge, Mass.: MIT Press, 1966, pp. 15–84.
   A long, difficult essay in which McNeill sketches in detail the history of early syntactic development.

SALUS, PETER. *Linguistics*. New York: Bobbs-Merrill, 1969.
    This is one of the more compact and readable treatments of the theory of grammar—a good place to start further reading. Available in paperback.
SLOBIN, DAN I. *Psycholinguistics*. Glenview, Ill.: Scott, Foresman, 1971.
    This book might be a good place to start your future reading. The two chapters about psycholinguistic principles and the chapter about language development go into more depth than this chapter, yet are still readable.

chapter 5

DEVELOPMENT OF SEMANTICS

One of the least understood aspects of children's development is how meanings come to be attached to language structure. The difficulty in discussing this problem is twofold: First, we do not understand the nature of the semantic system that the child is acquiring, and second, there has been very little research into the process of this acquisition.

WORDS AND OBJECTS

When we think about meaning, probably the first thing that comes to mind is the idea of "definition"—that is, the idea that words have referents in the real world, that words stand for things. We assume that the first words uttered by children are names of things. When the baby says "mama," the mother is happy because she believes the baby is using a label to indicate his recognition of her. Actually, as noted in Chapter 4, it is far more likely that the child's first words stand for sentences rather than objects. In other words, the baby may say "mama," and mean "Here is Mama," "Where is Mama?" "Come here, Mama," or "I see Mama." What "mama" means at any given time depends on the circumstances in which the word is uttered. The child begins to talk not with the adult dictionary in which words have meanings corresponding to entities in the world, but rather with a sentence dictionary in which each word corresponds to a number of sentences.

As the number of words in the child's vocabulary increases and as he encounters more situations in which the words can be used, the sentence dictionary becomes very cumbersome. At this point, the child begins to use individual words as meanings that can be combined into sentences. This is closer to the way adults use words, but it is still different. An adult thinks of words in terms of very limited, "dictionary" definitions. Children's word definitions are much less precise because the entries in their "dictionaries" are incomplete. For example, the child might know that "ball" refers to a spherical object that is thrown and have no idea that the word means something different in the sentence "Cinderella went to the ball." He might interpret this sentence to mean that Cinderella approached the round object. As another example, a child who heard the sentences "He called up his girl friend" and "He called up the stairs" might be willing to accept the sentence "He called up the stairs and his girl friend." In fact, McNeill (1965) found that children aged four to seven repeat meaningful sentences such as "The mouse ate the cheese" with no more efficiency than they repeat anomalous sentences such as "The string ate the cup." Eight-year-olds, however, repeat meaningful sentences much better than they repeat anomalous ones. Theoretically, the eight-year-old's dictionary entries are more complete, so he is able to use meaning to help him remember the meaningful sentence. To the younger child, one sentence is about as difficult as the other, because his store of semantic information is incomplete.

Further information about children's word meanings can be gained through word association experiments. In a word association test, the tester says a "prompt" word, and the subject says the first word that pops into his mind. Older children (eight and over) and adults usually say words (*associates*) of the same grammatical class as the prompt word; the associates will often be either the same or opposite in meaning. Responses of older children and adults to common words are quite predictable:

PROMPT	ASSOCIATION
dark	light
deep	shallow
rapid	fast

Younger children's associations are less consistent, and some are quite anomalous to adults:

PROMPT	ASSOCIATION
soft	wall
bright	rake

Others look like words that might be next to each other in sentences:

PROMPT	ASSOCIATION
deep	hole
dark	night

Perhaps younger children's associations are less predictable because their dictionary entries are incomplete. Adults may find younger children's responses strange because the child's word meanings (and thus his word associations) are not like those of adults.

To summarize, the child seems to go through three stages in acquiring meanings for words. First, each word seems to mean an entire sentence. Next, words have meanings, but the meanings are less complete and specific than adult meanings. Finally, adult meanings are learned. We know little about what causes the change from stage one to stage two, except that having words mean whole sentences is a cumbersome system and the child seems to recognize its basic inefficiency. The change from stage two to stage three is more gradual (although there is a big change around eight years of age). The change seems to come about through the adding of more and more specific additions to a word's definition.

Which leads us back to the question: What is in a word's definition? What form does the dictionary in our head take? It seems to take the form of rules, just as phonology and the syntax parts of language do. But in semantics we have only the barest inkling of what the rules are like. The rules seem to be of two types. First, there are *markers,* which go with each word and together add up to its meaning—just as the distinctive features of a sound add up to how it is pronounced. Second, there are *selection restrictions,* which are rules telling in what places the word may be used with consistent meaning.

The set of semantic markers that go with a particular word corresponds in some ways to the dictionary definition of that word. For example, the semantic markers of "dog" might include "furry," "four legs," "barks," "wagging tail." The acquisition of the set of semantic markers for a given word may be described as a process of *concept* development.

As Quine (1964) has expressed it, the child who is developing concepts must develop *individuated* terms. To develop individuated terms, the child must have some conception of the permanency of recurring objects. He must realize that the moon he sees in the sky tonight is the same moon that was there last night and that there are not two moons, or sixty. Alternatively, he must realize that the apple he eats for lunch is not the same apple he ate for lunch yesterday, but another apple. The child does not truly use individuated terms until he can understand the difference between "that apple," "not that apple," "an apple," "some apple," "another apple," "these apples." In this sense, it could be said that the child's word "mama" does not become a label for his mother until he learns the difference between "my mama," "not my mama," "my mama in a different dress," and so forth. To say that the child understands these various uses of a word implies that the child has developed a *concept* to go with a certain label.

Saying that a child has developed a correspondence between label and concept is quite different from saying that he has developed a correspondence between label and thing. When we speak of the concept "chair," for instance, we are not speaking of one particular chair, but rather of some quality of "chairness" that is shared by and unique to all chairs. The child must develop a set of working concepts before he can properly classify all the objects in his world. It is often easy to observe the progress of this development in children's speech. For example, a young friend named Andrew began his attempt with the word "car." This word was first applied only to the family Volkswagen, indicating a very narrow sense of "car." After a time, Andrew began to apply the word to all cars, trucks, and tractors, and soon he was using it to label anything that moved on wheels. At this point, Andrew's concept of "car" was too broad. It needed to be refined. He soon learned to distinguish trucks and used the word "tuck" to label these. Later he used the word "bus" to label another set of vehicles. This is exactly like the process of overgeneralization and differentiation we see in the child's learning of the sound system and the rules of syntax.

The point here is that Andrew had to learn that not all moving things with wheels are called by one word. He had to learn which of these things could be properly grouped together under one label. It is not so easy to put the meaning of the concept "car" into words so that it can be distinguished from truck or bus. The child seems to develop such concepts by trial and error —through experience with the environment.

The development of selection restrictions, however, is not so easy to observe. We know that when selection restrictions are violated, anomalous sentences such as "The paper eats the dog's dinner" result. The semantic features of the word "paper" do not match the selection restrictions of the word "eat." "Eat" is a verb that is used with animate nouns, and "paper" does not include the semantic marker "animate." The word "bark," in one of its senses, has semantic features that match the selection restrictions of the word "tree," so we can talk about "the bark on the oak tree." However, in another sense of the word "bark," the semantic features match the selection features of the word "dog," and cannot be associated with "tree" at all, as we do not talk about "how loudly the tree barks." It is the necessity for matching semantic features with selection restrictions that can cause problems for a child when he begins to use words in combination. If the concept that corresponds with a given word for the child does not contain all the necessary semantic features, then errors will occur when the child begins to use that word in combination with other words.

Unfortunately, this tells us nothing at all about how the child learns the selection restrictions for words. The one thing that seems clear is that this learning does not occur until the child starts to combine words to make sentences.

DEVELOPMENT OF SENTENCE MEANINGS

Up to this point, we have discussed only individual words. Selection restrictions operate within sentence structures, but only affect individual words. Yet when you put words together to make a sentence, you make a statement—a total sentence meaning, which is somehow more than the sum of its parts. The "total sentence meaning" is evaluated by speakers and listeners. For example, we would not readily accept the sentence "The paper bit the car" because such an event is unlikely in the extreme. The sentence would be regarded as odd by a listener, even though the structure is perfectly adequate.

As the example above indicates, when we analyze a sentence, we have to look at meaning as well as structure. This is especially true of children's speech because structural description alone does not always give a full picture of what the child said. Bloom (1971) argues that the structural description of children's two-word sentences as "pivot structures" (see Chapter 4) is inadequate because it fails to take semantics into account. For example, she observed the sentence "Mommy sock" being said twice by a child in one day's observations. The pivot-grammar linguist would have treated both sentences as the same event. But in one case the child was picking up his mother's sock (*Mommy's sock* —possessive), and in the other the mother was putting the child's sock on the child (*Mommy's putting on my sock*—descriptive). It is possible to think of several more situations in which "Mommy sock" might occur. The child might pick up one of his father's socks in the presence of his mother (*Mommy, here's a sock*), or he might bring the mother his own sock—either to identify it (*Mommy, this is my sock*) or to ask the mother to help him put it on (*Mommy, put on my sock*). If you take only syntax into account, all these instances of "Mommy sock" look the same. Yet they are five distinct speech events, as attention to the semantic dimension reveals. Eventually, it will be necessary for the child to learn the structural alternatives available to him for expressing all these different meanings. How the child comes to associate various structures with their total meanings is unclear.

The moral of this story is that when a child speaks, listeners should take into account what the child means as well as what he says. Given how little we know about semantics, this can be a very difficult task.

✳SUMMARY✳

We know little about semantics because we have no unifying theory to explain it in the sense that distinctive features explain phonology, for example. We have discovered that word meanings seem to develop in three stages: First, words have entire-sentence meanings. Second, with grammatical speech (about age two to three) words have incomplete definitions. Third (at around age seven to eight), words take on adult-like definitions.

Markers are rules that specify word meaning. Selection restrictions describe in what positions a word may be used. We do not know the precise form of either of these types of rules. When a solid semantic theory comes along, it will probably make hypotheses about the forms of these rules.

In addition to studying the meanings of individual words, we must attend to the total meanings of sentences. This is especially important in children's speech because the same two-word sentence may have several meanings.

Read This

BLOOM, LOIS. "Why Not Pivot Grammars?" *Journal of Speech and Hearing Disorders,* 36 (Feb. 1971), 40–50.

Bloom's criticism of pivot grammars is that they do not give enough information about what the child knows. She advocates paying greater attention to the child's semantic system.

BROWN, ROGER. *Words and Things.* New York: Free Press, 1958.

An easy-to-read and interesting account of what we mean by "meaning."

MCNEILL, DAVID. "Semantic Development, *The Acquisition of Language.* New York: Harper & Row, 1970, chap. 8.

This chapter provides a psycholinguistic approach to the problem of how children develop semantic systems.

chapter 6

DEVELOPMENT OF PRAGMATICS

> Not grammar, but the act of speech is the core and starting
> point of description of the place of language in human life.

Thus does anthropologist Dell Hymes (1969) ask us to analyze
how man *uses* his language, quite apart from the structure or
content of the language system itself. A focus upon patterns of
usage, upon "pragmatics," is an especially important aspect of the
child's communicative development.

Looking at child speech from this perspective requires us to
ask the questions: What is the child doing to communicate? How
do details of his linguistic and extralinguistic codes enter into
actual speaking and listening situations? In short, we are investi-
gating the child's learning of the rules of social interaction
within his community.

Sociologists and anthropologists frequently have discussed the
fact that men respond to social situations in ways that can be described by rules similar to rules of language. Let us illustrate by
example: Two American adult males acquainted with each other
meet on the street. It is easy to predict that the things they say to
each other will be brief, both will speak, and the likelihood of
such words as "hi" or "hello" is extremely high.

In every kind of communication situation we meet in a day,
we are aware that the dynamics of that situation affect us. If we
step into an elevator, we are usually silent and look at the floor
indicator. On a first date with a "nice girl" we confine conversation to politics and weather, with only oblique references to why
we are participating in the encounter. In all probability, you do

not tell off-color jokes if you are speaking to your grandmother. You are aware of the rules of social interaction. All these varieties of situations make demands on the kind of language we use. The fact that we consistently follow them is evidence that we are aware of these rules of usage inherent in situations—just as your ability to do a passive transformation in Chapter 3 indicates your implicit knowledge of linguistic rules.

The relationship between rules of grammar and rules of usage is like that between the rules of a game such as chess and the strategies (tactics) that allow you to be a good player (see Eric Berne's *Games People Play*). You can learn the rules of chess in just a few minutes: how each piece moves, what constitutes a checkmate, and so forth. But at this point you are a very poor player: You know nothing about what to do in actual playing situations. That takes longer to learn than the rules and usually requires a great deal of practice. Similarly, a child learns most of the rules of grammar in just a few months. But this does not mean that he is a mature speaker. It is only after several years' experience with various speech situations that his patterns of usage resemble those of adults. Learning to speak appropriately is like learning how to play chess well. There is no end to the task; it continues throughout life.

Although learning pragmatics is a lifelong task, children do show awareness of it at an early age. Even a very small child speaks differently to his friends than to his parents. He speaks in still different manners when addressing his baby brother, his teddy bear, his imaginary playmate. He also speaks differently to the same people under different circumstances. How he speaks to his mother during a meal, for instance, is different from how he speaks when they are playing together, and either of these situations can be varied still further by such factors as the child's imminent need to go to the bathroom or his guilt over having stolen from the cookie jar.

If you look at his speech to measure how the child adjusts his speech to situations, you may still often use the tools of linguistics discussed in Chapters 3 through 5. The difference is that now we are concerned less with details of linguistics themselves and more with how these details are used to meet the demands of particular features of the situation. One procedure for figuring out how children are reacting to situations is something like this:

1. Determine what the linguistic demands of a particular situation are. For example, if I ask you a question that begins with "why," I expect an answer that begins with "because." This is a rule of English usage. If you ask me: "Where are you going?" and I respond "Yes," you will be confused (and rightly so).

2. Now that you know how *adults* react to such situations, put children of various ages in similar situations and see how they react. This gives you an opportunity to examine their pragmatic development, just as we examined syntax development in Chapter 3.

In addition to setting up various demands for linguistic usage, communication situations also set up demands that we use speech to perform certain *tasks*. For example, an answer to a question can be perfect grammatically, yet still make little sense. Suppose I asked you:

> "Why did you eat my cookie?"

and you responded:

> "Because my mommy said that we are going to buy a house in the country."

Your answer is grammatical, but it is of no help to me because it makes no sense in terms of my question. This also works the other way: You can communicate without obeying grammar rules. Suppose that to my same question you had replied:

> "Hungry."

You have not really used all available grammatical tools, but I could at least understand the answer to my question.

These two situational demands may be described as *demands of grammar* (what grammatical forms are called for in the situation) and *demands of function* (what verbal tasks must be performed in the situation). It is sometimes important to keep these two aspects separate.

Hopper (1971) examined children's responses to questions such as those above and found differences between four-year-olds and five-year-olds in meeting demands of function, but not in meeting demands of grammar. For example, to the question "Why do you write with a pencil?" a four-year-old might say: "Because, I . . . um . . . just do." A five-year-old might say: "Because it's better than a crayon." This led Hopper to hypothesize that speech development during the fifth year of life centers around learning to meet demands of function. This fits with the research (see Chapter 4) that has shown that syntax is largely developed by about age four.

Learning to talk is a dynamic interplay between learning bits of grammar and bits of appropriate usage (function). These two kinds of learning are not independent of each other. A child uses a rule of grammar only when he figures out a use for it. Whether he "knows" that piece of grammar is a rather academic distinction if you are the parent or teacher of a child who is failing in school. For these reasons, a strategy of confronting a child with situations requiring particular speech behavior may be the best method of instruction for the closely tied together skills of grammar and function. This idea underlies many potential educational innovations; we shall return to it in Chapter 9.

ASPECTS OF SITUATIONAL CONTEXT

Up to this point, we have been discussing how to study child speech within the matrix of the communication situation. The major point throughout has been that neither adults nor children speak the same way all the time, and much variation is due to the constraints of communication situations. Now we examine the internal dynamics of communication situations—to ask what aspects of situations are important in shaping speech behavior and the child's speech development.

We shall discuss five aspects of situational context that make demands upon how a person communicates. These aspects of situational context are:

1. the people present
2. what was said just before
3. the topic of conversation

4. the task that communication is being used to accomplish
5. the times and places in which the communication occurs

With each of these elements of situational context, we shall discuss briefly the effects upon adult speech and then focus upon how they enter into the scheme of the child's speech development.

The People Present: Personal Context

It is obvious that the people who are in any situation shape that situation and have effects upon communication. If you hear a spicy dirty joke, which you are dying to tell someone, you have the sense to wait for an appropriate audience. You do not tell it to your mother or the checkout girl at the grocery. If you are a teacher furious with your principal, you will express yourself differently to the principal himself than to a co-teacher. We make adjustments in our speaking behavior according to our audience hundreds of times a day—almost without ever thinking about it.

Children, however, have to learn this skill. So your four-year-old is likely to say innocently, when being introduced to your boss: "My dad says you're an old tightwad." Still, that same four-year-old already has developed great skill in speaking to his playmates—using jargon and sentence structures that you rarely hear. You rarely hear them because the first time he said "Mommy, you smell funny" at the dinner table, you chewed him out—teaching him some things about personal context.

Research about child speech has usually overlooked the personal context dimension. Thus children in nursery schools and kindergartens are often tested by strange (to the child) adults (often men, while teachers are usually women). This can be frightening to a child, which probably explains why children often speak so little in such contexts, even though they can be seen jabbering on the playground before and after. We should be careful to recall at such times that a child often knows things he does not say at any single time.

An even more unfortunate situation sometimes occurs with minority children. Imagine a five-year-old black child who rarely sees a white person and for whom any white person is probably an object to be feared. Suppose then that someone from the local university (well-dressed white male) comes around to give him a "language advancement test" of one kind or another. The child, in this fear-arousing personal context, will say very little. The researcher then publishes a research report on delayed language in disadvantaged children—based on the language behavior of children in this unique and (to the child) threatening situation.

One point that can be gained from this is: When you are analyzing anything a child says, it can be important to ask yourself to whom the child was speaking. Conversely, when looking at how a child responds to someone else's speech, it is wise to ask who the speaker was—for that may be as much the cause of the child's response as what is said.

Finally, if you are in charge of a classroom, the kind of person you are has great effects on the behavior of your students. Teachers who stress authority and discipline often create entire classrooms of sullen, hostile, uncommunicative children. Teachers who openly encourage an atmosphere free from fear may find students more responsive.

What Has Been Said Before: Message Context

Often we tend to look at a single sentence "out of context." Suppose you are a movie critic and you write this sentence about a movie: "Despite flashes of brilliant acting, this was a horribly dull film." Then the next day's paper carries an ad for the movie attributing to you the phrase "brilliant acting," as though it were a plug for the movie. You would claim that you had been quoted out of context.

What goes before (and after, too) can be just as important in conversation. Consider these two examples:

1. You are a teacher, and your principal calls you into his office. His face is red, his eyes flashing. In his hand he holds your lesson plan for the month. "You can't use these books," he sputters. "The board of education would have my job. *Sometimes I wonder what you use for brains.*"

2. As you walk by the principal's office, he shouts: "Hey, your shoelace is untied!" You stop to look and he chortles "April

Fool!" You are mildly embarrassed as he says: "It's four o'clock in the afternoon, and you are still forgetting what day this is. *Sometimes I wonder what you use for brains."*

In both of these examples, the same person sits at the same desk and says the same (italicized) sentence to you. Yet your reaction is likely to be very different in the two situations. This difference is due to the context set up by other sentences immediately preceding the one we are analyzing.

We know little about how and when the child learns the importance of conversational context. But this is one area in which schools could help. Perhaps workbooks could be developed in which paragraphs are missing one sentence, and the child could get a feel for conversational context by filling in the missing sentence. Perhaps tapes setting a situation could be played, and children could discuss "what happens next."

The Topic Being Discussed: Content Context

Anyone who knows children knows that the topic being discussed makes a lot of difference in what they say. Some children who rarely say a cogent word in response to questions on IQ tests will deliver concise and eloquent statements on the subjects of baseball or anatomical differences between boys and girls. All people of all ages prefer to talk about things they are interested in.

Try taking an interesting machine—say, a carousel slide projector—into a nursery school or kindergarten. Sit down in one corner during a free-play time, turn it on, and begin to show slides against a wall. In two minutes, children will be all around you, asking questions, begging to operate the machine, generally causing a commotion. Such gimmicks can be an almost unending source of topics of conversation even for children who talk little.

Educational practices often fail to take into account what sorts of topics for discussion would motivate students. Teaching methods designed without appreciation of this situational dimension often fall upon deaf student ears. In *How Children Learn,* John Holt describes how schools would probably teach children to speak if given that assignment: First, the children would be taught to make all the phonemes, next how to combine these sounds into words, then how to combine the words into syntactic patterns—all by sheer memory. Only *after* the child had mastered all this would teachers tell children some ways speech can be used, or what some words mean. This example may sound far-fetched, but many of our teaching methods have no tie-ins with matters of interest to the students. In a sense, this is what the modern call for "relevance" in education is all about. Children want to discuss matters that touch on their interests in some way, that fit into their content context. This does not mean, obviously, that children cannot be encouraged to be interested in new things. It is simply an attempt to point out that children are not likely to talk much about things that *don't* interest them.

The Goal: Task Context

In looking at any utterance, it is useful to ask: What is the speaker trying to do? What kind of discourse is he trying to generate, what objectives is he trying to accomplish? When you say to your child: "Would you please take out the garbage?" it is important to realize that, in spite of the grammatical structure of the sentence, you are *not* asking a question. You are giving an order. If the child's response is not "proper" (obedience), you realize that he has broken a pragmatic rule. (As with most pragmatic and linguistic rules, we notice the presence of a rule most when it is broken. Other times we don't think about it.)

Research has shown that listeners can make subtle distinctions about what communication tasks are being set for them when they are asked various kinds of questions. Williams and Naremore (1969) studied the responses of fifth-grade children to three orders of questions:

1. Simple (requiring only a yes / no response):
   "Do you play baseball?"
2. Naming (require a single-word label):
   "What games do you play?"
3. Elaboration (can only be answered by a sentence or more description or elaboration):
   "How do you play baseball?"

The researchers found that children consistently fulfilled the demands of these question situations. Further, they found that middle-class children tended to elaborate even in situations that did not specifically require it. These findings prompted them to speculate that the often-found communication differences between different social classes may be primarily in the area of how language is used rather than in the sphere of linguistic development. Hopper (1971) constructed quasiexperimental situations by asking four- and five-year-old children questions similar to those used by Williams and Naremore. Even children this young showed remarkable abilities to respond according to the demands of question situations.

In looking at children's speech it can often be helpful to ask the question: What is the child trying to do? To answer this question, you must examine the situation from the child's point of views. To show how this can be helpful, suppose your child said:

> "Daddy shirt."

It is most tempting to assume that he is pointing to a shirt belonging to Daddy ("Daddy's shirt"). But suppose also that the child is holding a shirt of his *own*. Then you might think he is saying "Daddy, here's my shirt." But suppose that he is holding the shirt up with an impelling look on his face and that he is wearing no shirt. Then you know he is saying "Daddy, put on my shirt."

How do you know all this? By intuition, the same way you know about grammar rules. If you are often around children, you can usually tell what they are talking about. It is especially easy to interpret what a child says because it is usually directly related to what he is doing. Children often accompany actions with descriptions:

> "I'm gonna go outside now."

These facts all make it easier to interpret child speech from the viewpoint of what task the child is doing. If parents and teachers force themselves to examine child speech in the light of content context, many misunderstandings can be avoided.

This focus on what the child is doing can also help us avoid what might be called the *grammar fetish*. We are guilty of the grammar fetish when we correct a child's grammar even though we can understand him perfectly well:

Johnny: Hitler were a great man.
Teacher: No, Johnny, Hitler *was* a great man.

Obviously this teacher has missed the boat. Yet there is a bit of this teacher in all of us—an instinctive urge to correct grammar. If we are careful to examine children's speech in terms of task context, we will often be less concerned with details of grammar and more concenred with sane and decent content.

Time and Place: Surrounding Physical Context

Labov (1970a) suspected that black children were not performing well on language tasks out of fear of the interviewer, so he undertook a study using a black fieldworker who knew the children being tested. Results were still bad. So the fieldworker dressed less formally, sat on the floor with the children, and opened a bag of potato chips. In this situation, the children were happy to talk, and a successful interview was conducted.

This example accents the importance of the physical context in which communication takes place. It is obvious that some people are more comfortable and talkative in certain circumstances than in others. If your principal comes to your classroom, you may be less nervous than if he asks to see you in his office.

Children are even more sensitive to physical context than adults are, and they also use it more in their communication. They are, of course, apprehensive about new environments. They often are very quiet for their first half hour in a strange house. When returning home from such a place, children (obviously relieved) sometimes talk a great deal.

Surrounding physical context affects child speech in another respect, which is at once subtle yet more pervasive than the large-scale changes in the scene we have discussed. That is the extent to which children use context in early attempts to communicate. A child of about fourteen months can indicate objects and food he wants by pointing and grunting—without saying a word.

Even after children learn to talk, they still make heavy use of context—showing things, pointing, and so forth—in communication situations. The example used earlier about the child saying "Daddy shirt" illustrates this.

Children also use context in understanding sentences. Try saying this sentence to a three-year-old:

> "The elephant was kissed by the bear."

Then ask him who is doing the kissing, and he will be confused. Usually the actor in a sentence is the first noun, so he may guess the elephant; yet he will know there is something queer about this sentence. He will act unsure. If you present the same sentence and ask the same question while showing the child a picture of a bear kissing an elephant on the cheek, he can answer easily.

If you want to see how heavily the three-year-old depends on surrounding physical context, try this trick: Provide the same sentence, ask the same question, but show the child a picture of an elephant kissing a bear. He will be more confused than ever, and will almost always give a response agreeing with the picture.

This activity (an unending source of amusement for experimenters) also works with other kinds of questions. Hold up a glass of water in front of a child of age three and ask: "What do you do with a spoon?" About half the time the response will be, "You drink with it."

Similar alterations of visual context can fool even older children. Carol Chomsky (1969) showed children a doll wearing a blindfold and asked: "Is this doll easy to see or hard to see?" Children of about age five or six usually replied that the doll was hard to see; they were tricked by visual context.

These examples show how young children often use visual context as a "crutch" to help them interpret sentences using hard-to-understand grammar rules. This suggests devising teaching strategies that use context to help children master grammar. Playing with dolls and describing their actions, for example, could provide an almost endless source of contexts to aid comprehension of difficult sentences.

NONVERBAL COMMUNICATION

The visual context that children use to interpret messages they hear is often in the form of facial expression or other manifestations of nonverbal communication. At an early age, children demonstrate remarkable facility both in understanding and creating nonverbal communication.

The child's first attempts to communicate are mostly nonverbal. The first smile, which usually occurs at about age one month, is certainly a kind of communication. When a toddler wants something, he usually signals his desire by pointing or some other nonverbal gesture. Dependence upon such methods continues even after the child can speak. A three-year-old is more likely to point and say: "I want somma dat," than to name the object he desires.

The development of nonverbal systems of communication seems to parallel that of the verbal ones. As children gain greater facility with speech, they also learn to use greater varieties of gestures and facial expression. By adulthood, speakers have attained remarkable nonverbal expressive abilities (though use of these abilities is largely subconscious). Minute changes of eyebrow positions or small variations in the way the corners of the mouth turn come to have correlations with the verbal system; in effect, they come to stand for meanings in much the same way that words do.

Although the nonverbal communication system is sophisticated and useful, it seems narrower in scope than the verbal system. Used mostly in communicating *emotions,* it is of little help in cognitive tasks such as problem solving and discussing abstract concepts. It is these latter abilities that make man's verbal communication system so different from those of other animals. The nonverbal communication system is less unique; other primates seem to communicate nonverbally about as effectively as men do.

We should not regard the limitations of nonverbal communication as reasons to avoid its study. Children are quite adept at it, and its use can aid both their verbal abilities and their general expressive capacities. The difficulty many adults experience in verbally expressing emotions is rarely found in children (who are aided by practice in nonverbal communicating). Perhaps if we recognized the value of such nonverbal expression—rather than constantly emphasizing the cognitive and academic—we could avoid some of the many communication problems that arise when we fail to read accurately the nonverbal cues available to us.

SUMMARY

It is important to examine how children speak in response to usage demands imposed by communication situations. One way to approach this aspect of child speech is to examine various aspects of speech situations to which adults regularly react and then to study children's development toward adult usage. Five aspects of communication situations were discussed: (1) the people present, (2) the surrounding utterances, (3) the topic of conversation, (4) the task being performed, and (5) the physical setting in which the communication occurs.

Read This

CAZDEN, COURTNEY. "The Neglected Situation in Child Language Research and Education," in Frederick Williams (ed.), *Language and Poverty*. Chicago: Markham, 1970, pp. 81–101.

Cazden discusses the need for more study of the effects of situations on child speech, reviews research that relates to situation variables, and makes suggestions. Quite readable.

HOPPER, ROBERT. "Expanding the Notion of Competence," *The Speech Teacher*, XX (January 1971), 29–35.

This article advocates analyzing child speech from the viewpoint of usage and demonstrates several advantages of such an approach.

HYMES, DELL. *On Communicative Competence.* Philadelphia: University of Pennsylvania Press, 1970.

A more detailed treatment of the need for study of situational variables in all communication research.

WILLIAMS, FREDERICK, and RITA C. NAREMORE. "On the Functional

Analysis of Social Class Differences in Modes of Speech," *Speech Monographs,* XXXVI (June 1969), 77–102.

This article reports results of analyses of speech of upper- and lower-class elementary-school children. The authors outline a scheme of "modes of speech" to explain parallel development of grammar and usage.

chapter 7

THOUGHT AND SPEECH

The major chicken-and-egg question in children's communication is this: Which comes first, thinking or talking? Obviously, thought and speech are closely intertwined. How the two are related is much less obvious. Here are the major possibilities:

1. *Speech shapes thought.* The course of communicative development molds the child's general cognitive and perceptual processes.

2. *Thought shapes speech.* Communicative development is simply one aspect of cognitive development. It is not the child's speech that molds his thinking, but rather it is the development of thinking that causes communicative development.

It is important to decide which of these views best reflects the relationship between thinking and speaking because this decision dictates how you teach the child. If speech shapes thought, then instruction should center upon verbal methods. If thinking shapes language, then cognitive tasks should aid communication development.

DEVELOPMENT OF THINKING

In order to discuss relationships between thought and speaking, we must examine how thinking develops in children. We owe most of what we know about child thought to the research of the French psychologist Jean Piaget. According to Piaget, child thought progresses through three basic stages. The child at birth is totally *autistic,* or centered upon himself. Between (roughly) ages three to seven, children are *egocentric* in their thinking, which means they are still somewhat self-centered but less so than in the period of autistic thought. Finally, the child begins to think in a *socialized* manner, more like adults.

Autistic Thought

The very young child's thought is autistic. Autistic thought works through images, fantasy, and imagination. Autistic thought is self-centered to the point that the child does not even think of himself as separate from the rest of the world.

How the child feels at this stage is anyone's guess because the child himself can't tell us about it. Piaget guesses that in the autistic phase the child sees no particular connections among events around him. Only slowly does he realize that the person who feeds him today is the same mother who fed him yesterday. Until this time, the mother "does not exist" for the child except when he can see her. It is no help for a mother to say "I'll be back" until the child realizes that she exists when she is out of his sight. Further, Piaget guesses that during this phase the child is mostly interested in his physical sensations and the results of moving his arms, legs, and so on. It is for this reason that Piaget calls the period of autistic thought the *sensori-motor* stage of development.

Egocentric Thought

Somewhere around age two, the child begins to make clear distinctions between himself as an individual and the rest of the world. Harried mothers call this period the "terrible twos" because of the child's uncooperativeness. Piaget would call it the beginnings of the period of *egocentric thought*.

The egocentric child knows he is an individual, he knows speech is used for communication, and he knows thinking can solve problems. What he does not know is *how*—how he is different, how he can communicate using speech, how he can figure out proper solutions to problems.

One major reason for this lack of communicating and problem-solving strategies is simple inexperience. The child sees people reaching conclusions but knows little about the reasoning behind the conclusions. Thus he "reaches conclusions" himself without going through any real reasoning process. A little later he realizes that there must be reasons for conclusions, but almost any "pseudoreason" will do:

> Adult: I'm going to spank you.
> Child: Don't spank me because I have Kleenex in my pocket.
>
> Adult: Why is this called a handkerchief?
> Child: Because my mommy ties it around my head when the wind blows.
>
> Adult: Why did the balloon break?
> Child: Because it couldn't hold its breath.

In addition to this simple inexperience, the egocentric child is tightly *tied to his own perceptual point of view.* He knows that other people exist, but assumes they see things just as he does. Consider this conversation between Brian and his mother:

> Mother: What is Kenny's mommy's name?
> Brian: Mrs. Myers.
> Mother: What is Adam's mommy's name?
> Brian: Mrs. Black.
> Mother: What is your mommy's name?
> Brian: *Mommy!*
> Mother: What do other children call me?
> Brian: Mommy.
> Mother: No, other children call me Mrs. . . .
> Brian: Mommy.
> Mother: What is my last name?
> Brian: Hopper.
> Mother: Then children call me Mrs. . . .
> Brian: Mommy.

In this case, Brian knows the formula for calling a mother "Mrs. ———," but cannot apply this to his own mother. He cannot see his own mother from the point of view of another child.

Children are just as tightly tied to their visual point of view. If you ask a three-year-old to show you a picture he is holding, he will show it to himself—on the assumption that you will also be able to see. The egocentric child lacks "role-taking ability"—he cannot put himself in another's shoes.

As a result, the child's thinking and talking are largely based upon what he can see. For example, four-year-olds usually believe nickels are more valuable than dimes because they are bigger.

A third aspect of egocentric thought is the use of oversimplified concepts. *The egocentric child is only able to think about one aspect of a situation at a time,* so some of his concepts are different from those of adults.

You can demonstrate how children think in terms of one aspect of a situation by trying one of Piaget's famous "conservation" experiments. *Conservation* is the ability to judge that when you have a certain amount of a substance and put it in a container of a different shape, you still have the same amount. In concrete terms, here is what you do.

First, you pour water into two identical containers, having a child (between four and seven) tell you when the amount of water in the containers is exactly the same. Typically, children make this judgment by observing the height of the water in the containers. At this point, you have two containers with quantities of water judged by the child to be equal:

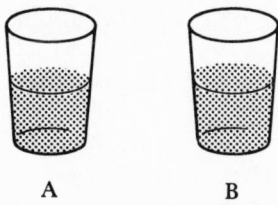

A   B

Next, you take container B and pour its water into a tall thin container, giving the following situation:

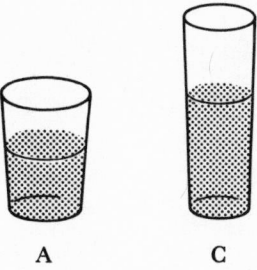

A   C

Now you ask the child: "Do we still have the same amount of water in each glass, or does one glass have more?" The child almost always replies that the tall thin glass has more. He is paying attention to only one aspect of the situation: container height. He is ignoring width, which is also a factor. He seems to be operating according to a perceptual rule: The highest one has more.

If you pour the water from the tall thin container into the shorter fatter one, the child will again assert that the quantities are equal. One child, on being asked how it could be that the quantities could change when no water was added or taken away, answered tranquilly: "It's magic."

You can play a similar trick by making two rows of six checkers (or pennies)—one row spread apart and one close together:

(a)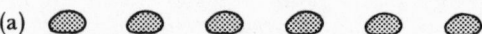

(b)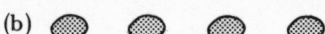

The "bigger" row will be judged by three- and four-year-olds to have more members. Five- and six-year-olds, who can count well, usually do not fall for this one.

These conservation experiments have been popular with researchers studying four- to seven-year-olds for several years. Mehler and Bever (1967) tried a conservation task with three-year-olds and made a startling discovery. They used two rows of clay lumps, one row having six members and the other having four.

(a)

(b)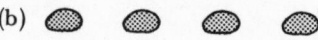

Ordinarily, all children can tell that row (a) has more. But if you push row (a) closer together,

(a)

(b)

four- and five-year-olds will say row (b) has more. They follow the rule "bigger means more" and are fooled. Mehler and Bever's remarkable finding was that *two-year-olds were not fooled!* They correctly chose row (a) as having more. This means that the younger, less egocentric children had not yet learned the "bigger means more" rule. In everyday life, the older egocentric child makes pretty good judgments using this rule, but in conservation experiments he is fooled. It is not until about age five or six, when he learns to count, that the child stops misjudging in this experiment. This suggests that "inability to conserve" is not a general part of immaturity (because in some instances very young children do conserve), but rather it is part of the egocentric thought stage.

THINKING AND TALKING

Now we are ready to consider how speaking abilities and thinking abilities are related in communication development.

Speech Shapes Thought

It has been argued that language is not merely a means of expression, but also a kind of mold, which shapes the mind of the speaker. The words and sentence structures you use affect how you see your world (Whorf, 1956). In this view, the differences among languages represent differences in how speakers of those languages see the world. For example, Eskimoes have a large number of terms that would translate into English as "snow"; some refer to soft slushy snow, others to little cold flakes, still others to hardened snow in a glacier. Because we do not have names for these different kinds of snow, we cannot perceive them as clearly as Eskimoes do. For another example, suppose some culture had only one word to represent the colors blue and green (just as we use *blue* to cover shades from aqua to navy). Speakers from such a culture would have a hard time distinguishing differences among shades of blue and green because language would hamper them.

Whorf's view is supported by the fact that languages use different words, but it cannot account for the ways in which languages are alike (see Chapter 2). In short, although one's culture affects one's outlook, there is little evidence that the development of language per se is important to development of thought.

However, there is a related sense in which children's speech affects their thinking. Children often seem to *guide* their actions and thoughts with speech. A child often seems to "describe" what he is doing:

> "Now I'll draw a pig. . . and here's a place for him to live."

This use of speech has no communicative function. The child is not talking to anyone; he is simply guiding his actions with speech. Similarly, children can only add two numbers together by saying them out loud. We all use speech at some time or other to help us guide our thinking. A child or adult "in concentration" often moves his lips as he tries to solve a difficult problem. Finally, both adults and children often ask themselves questions to solve cognitive problems—another instance of speech guiding thought.

If any of these uses of speech aid thought development, then we ought to be able to teach concepts to children through training in speaking. Hermina Sinclair-de-Zwart (1969) examined children's performance on conservation tasks (like those described above) and tried to train children to do better on these kinds of tasks by asking questions about them. She found that there were no basic differences in overall linguistic ability between "conservers" and "nonconservers," although conservers used more comparative terms (e.g., "more" or "less") to describe the situations and nonconservers used absolute terms (e.g., "a lot" or "a little"). Sinclair-de-Zwart then taught the use of comparative terms to the nonconservers. She experienced no difficulty in teaching the forms to the children, but afterward the children did no better on the conservation task than they had in the first place. The conclusion is that knowing the linguistic forms used with advanced thinking does not make children more capable of doing the advanced thinking. Language is not the source of logic, but on the contrary, seems structured by logic.

Thought Shapes Speech

Piaget has long felt that language is part of a much larger complex of process thinking. His earliest research (in the 1920s) concentrated upon speech, but his later work examines more generalized cognitive processing. This emphasis is based on the assumption that how a child thinks is a dominant influence upon how he talks. Through his work and that of other researchers, it is becoming evident that this assumption is accurate.

It is even becoming clear that the three phases of thinking discussed in this chapter are associated with three kinds of strategies for sentence processing (Bever, 1970). The young autistic child's handling of sentences is intuitive, the egocentric child's sentence handling is closely tied to his perceptions, and only with the beginning of adult thought patterns is mature sentence processing possible.

INTUITIVE SENTENCE PROCESSING. The child does not begin speaking until near the end of the autistic phase of his thought, but he listens with comprehension well before he can talk. His handling of sentences during this period is like that of a naïve genius. There is no self-consciousness of what he is doing, yet he can understand most sentences he hears. At this stage, the child seems to understand the basic relationships between parts of a sentence in underlying structure. He comprehends, for example, that the noun phrase at the start of a sentence is "doing" the verb.

PERCEPTUAL SENTENCE PROCESSING. In the egocentric period, the child's handling of sentences, like his handling of conservation tasks, is closely tied to what he perceives. This "perceptual strategy" can be very helpful because many sentences that are meaningless to a younger child can be assigned meanings by the egocentric child—even though some of the meanings he assigns would make adults wince.

What happens is that the child uses semantics or context as a "crutch" to help him understand sentences with difficult structures. For example, if you said "The ice cream is eaten by the policeman," a five-year-old might not understand the structure of the sentence any better than a two-year-old. But the five-year-old will be able to figure out that something is eating and something is being eaten; this sentence has only one candidate for each of these because ice cream does not eat and policemen are not eaten. Thus, the five-year-old may be able to "guess" the correct meaning of this sentence. The same five-year-old, however, would have trouble with "The elephant was kissed by the bear" because this sentence is "reversible"—the elephant or the bear can be either kisser or kissed. The words in the sentence contain no semantic cues about which does the kissing. In this situation, the five-year-old's performance is little better than the three-year-old's.

Five-year-olds also get cues from context. If you show a five-year-old a picture of a bear kissing an elephant and say "The elephant was kissed by the bear," the child will be able to tell who did the kissing. You can tell he is depending upon context because if you show him a picture of the elephant doing the kissing and say the same sentence, his interpretation changes to agree with the picture.

This kind of sentence processing is tied to what the child perceives in the same way as are his interpretations of conservation tasks. It is not until about age eight, when he is outgrowing his egocentrism, that the child can decipher difficult sentences without being totally tied to the context in which the sentence is uttered.

SUMMARY

Development of thought processes influences communication development. The child passes through three stages of sentence processing, which correspond to the three major phases of his cognitive development.

The very young child thinks autistically and processes sentences intuitively. Children about three to seven think egocentrically and process sentences perceptually, using meanings of individual words and clues from context to help them decipher difficult sentence structures. Only with attainment of near-adult thinking patterns can children process difficult sentences as adults do.

Read This

FLAVELL, JOHN. *Communication and the Development of Role-Taking Skills in Children*. New York: Wiley, 1968.

Flavell explains well the development of abilities to "put yourself in their shoes" on the part of egocentric children.

FURTH, HANS G. *Piaget and Knowledge*. Englewood Cliffs, N. J.: Prentice-Hall, 1969.

All of Piaget's theorizing is collated in this book. Chapter 3, on language, is particularly good.

FURTH, HANS G. *Piaget for Teachers*. Englewood Cliffs, N. J.: Prentice-Hall, 1972.

A more readable and applied treatment of the same material covered in Furth's *Piaget and Knowledge*.

PIAGET, JEAN. *The Child's Conception of the World,* trans. Marjorie Wordon. New York: Harcourt Brace Jovanovich, 1928.

This book presents Piaget's ideas about how children structure their world. It contains many excellent examples of children's speech to illustrate points. As is true of all Piaget's writing, parts may be tough going, but it is worth dipping into.

PULASKI, MARY ANN SPENCER. *Understanding Piaget*. New York: Harper & Row, 1971.

Pulaski provides a simplified and highly readable summary of Piaget's ideas, with a focus on cognitive development rather than language per se. Many examples of children's speech are included.

PART THREE

chapter 8

HOW CHILDREN LEARN
TO COMMUNICATE

In Chapters 3 through 7, we discussed several aspects of communicative development. It was necessary to talk about each area in detail because each has its own terminology and because some phases of development take place in only one or a few of these areas. But communicative development is one organic growing process as much as it is many processes. This chapter brings together some communication acquisition processes that have generality across several of the specialized areas discussed in Part Two. The question we are asking is "How do children learn to talk?" In essence, we are looking for causes—for variables that bring about changes from babbling through child speech to adult speech.

BIOLOGY AND COMPETENCE

First, we restate the importance of the fact that human babies are born into a species of speaking animals. There is a strong biological predisposition toward developing implicit knowledge of linguistic (syntactic, phonological, semantic) relationships. That is just another way of saying that you are able to learn a language because you are human. You will also learn to *speak* a language —that is, you will learn the usage patterns of your community. We agree with Piaget that all this is a result of general processes of cognitive development: People learn to talk because that is part of learning to think as humans do.

This developmental emphasis highlights the ways in which all people are alike. Linguists like to say that each of us has a linguistic competence consisting of what we know about language. We would expand that concept to say that people possess *communicative competence,* covering knowledge of the entire range and scope of communication. This humanistic conception of communication encourages us to think that all men are brothers. We approve of that.

But as we look at the world around us, we see that some men are more brothers than others. We also see that even though we all have human intelligence, some men are smarter than others. Even though we all have communicative competence, some men communicate more effectively than others. All people are different as well as alike. A biological perspective on communication development explains how all men are alike, but not how each is different from every other man.

Children in the process of acquiring language share a common human birthright, but each child must face that process as an individual. Our theory of communicative development must take into account the dynamics of how the child encounters communication events, and how he learns.

Some early studies of grammar failed to do this. They built theories strictly on the basis of the internal workings of grammar. Researchers assumed that children would learn the "simplest" rules of grammar first and more complex varieties later. But when Bates (1967) predicted order of acquisition of some syntactic rules on the basis of complexity of the rules, results were directly the opposite of predictions. She concluded that the child's progress in language acquisition is more a result of his learning strategies than of the rules of grammar. We share this view, and the present chapter focuses largely upon the child's learning procedures.

Looking at learning strategies is especially important to educators, therapists, and parents because these people are all primarily concerned with why some children communicate more effectively than others. Several kinds of learning strategies children use to varying degrees in acquiring communication skills will be discussed in the next section.

LEARNING STRATEGIES

In Chapter 2, the controversy between rationalists and empiricists was analyzed. Our statement there that both the environment and the child's innate abilities are important for language learning must be reiterated here. In discussions of the strategies children employ in learning to talk, the dispute between those who emphasize the effects of the environment and those who emphasize the child's innate abilities or knowledge often generates more heat than light. We hope we can arrive at a reasonable resolution of this unprofitable controversy.

Operant Conditioning

The primary expression of empiricism can be found in the works of behavioral psychologist B. F. Skinner and his followers (most notably, Arthur Staats). The behaviorists argue that the kind of learning most important to the child's communicative development is operant conditioning. Operant conditioning occurs when a child's behavior results in some behavior from the environment, or some reaction within the child, which is reinforcing. The child's own internal responses or the behavior of other people will be reinforcing if they increase the probability that the child's behavior will occur again in circumstances similar to those in which it was reinforced. For example, if a child feels thirsty and says "wa wa" and is reinforced by getting a glass of water, the likelihood that he will say "wa wa" the next time he feels thirsty is increased. The critical part of this, or any other, operant conditioning situation is the reinforcement. The difficulty with the behaviorist approach lies in deciding, in a given situation, what was reinforcing and what was learned. For example, the behaviorists maintain that children learn to make grammatical sentences through a complex and delicately balanced combination of discriminative reinforcement in which certain of the child's language behaviors are reinforced and certain others are extinguished (because they are not reinforced). However, it is difficult to find any clear explanation of what kinds of behavior on the part of parents or others is reinforcement for the child's learning adult grammatical patterns. One possible (and obvious) reinforcement is praise for correct grammatical patterns and correction of incorrect patterns. However, there is some question as to how much correcting of grammar the average parent does, and what the child learns from it. For example, Brown and Hanlon (1970) argue that parents do not correct children on the basis of grammar. They found that when a child says a sentence that is true but ungrammatical, such as:

> "Mama isn't boy, he a girl"

his parents are likely to say: "That's right!" (which is reinforcement and should make children speak ungrammatically). But if the Walt Disney show is broadcast on Sunday, and the child says:

> "Walt Disney comes on Tuesday"

parents are likely to correct him, saying something like: "No, it comes on Sunday." According to Brown and Hanlon, parents of young children will reinforce sentences that are true and ungrammatical (but understandable) more often than sentences that are grammatical but wrong. Syntax cannot be learned by this kind of reinforcement alone and must be learned in some other way. This view makes sense when you consider how complex grammar is, yet how fast children pick it up. Even if it could be established that reinforcement plays a major role in children's learning of grammar, the question of how the child picked out grammatical sentences to say would remain open. Because a child cannot be reinforced in an operant conditioning situation until he emits some behavior, the question of how he comes to make his first grammatical sentences is important.

But syntax is not all that children must learn in order to communicate. The evidence that parents do reinforce sentence truth value indicates that operant conditioning may be an important learning strategy for acquiring knowledge about how sentences function within speech situations (pragmatics). A great deal about when to speak in what manner to whom is learned according to what modes of speech are reinforced. You learn not to swear around your mother from her reaction. You learn to compliment her dinner the same way. This may offer a hint to parents and teachers: You may be able to improve the things a child says by praising him when you are pleased, but years of teaching grammar by correction in the public schools should indicate that you are unlikely to improve his grammar solely by praising his good constructions or reacting negatively to his syntactic aberrations.

Imitation

One of the first characteristics of child speech noted by Brown and his associates is that much of what children say is in imitation of adult utterances. This imitation typically assumes the form of "telegraphic speech"—leaving out "functions" (inflections, auxiliary verbs, articles, prepositions, and conjunctions) and including high content words (nouns, verbs, and adjectives). The result looks like a telegram: interpretable but brief. If a parent says: "There's a red truck," the child is likely to say: "Red truck." Brown and Bellugi (1964) called this "imitation with reduction" and theorized that it was important to grammar learning. Even more important, they found that parents often "imitate" child utterances, expanding them by adding back the very words children are likely to leave out. This "imitation with expansion" seemed an efficient teaching device because it paired the child's immature sentence with the adult representation. As such, the parent's expansions could be regarded as a potent form of reinforcement.

But even though children and parents do imitate each other, it has never been proved that this imitating helps children learn to talk. In fact, Cazden (1965) found that language training using "imitation with expansion" produced little improvement in performance. Perhaps imitation, though a common event, is simply not an efficient enough learning strategy to explain much about communication development. Consider the following example: *

> Child: Nobody don't like me.
> Mother No, say "Nobody likes me."

* From David McNeill, "Developmental Psycholinguistics," in Frank Smith and George Miller (eds), *The Genesis of Language,* Cambridge, Mass.: MIT Press, 1966, p. 69.

Child: Nobody don't like me.

$\downarrow$

Eight repetitions of this dialogue.

$\downarrow$

Mother: No, now listen carefully;
         say "Nobody likes me."
Child: Oh! Nobody don't likes me.

The child finally *partially* corrected his utterance, so it is possible to teach through imitation. But for this case, at least, the process hardly seems very efficient.

The real importance of imitation to communicative development might be in learning the individual sounds and words of a language. Many times children will "play" with sounds, and often they will imitate with little regard for what a sentence means. Perhaps this play is important in learning about the sounds and words on which sentences are built. It is difficult to conceive of a child learning to use the proper word for any object in his environment except by imitating others.

Modeling

When Cazden (1965) tried to teach language to children using "imitation with expansion," she also employed (with a different group of children in the same experiment) a technique she called "modeling." Modeling teachers attempted never to repeat or expand child utterances; rather, they attempted to comment on what the child said—to answer questions, offer contributions on related topics, and so forth. In this way, the adult offered a model of mature speech for the child to emulate, without imitating.

Cazden found that the modeling training improved performance, while expansion, or imitating what the child said, did not. This leads to the hypothesis that children may learn some aspects of communication simply by "absorbing" and emulating sentences of adults they can hear speaking. This is a very tentative hypothesis. Cazden worked with a very small number of children. Also, her subjects were black and classified as economically deprived. This one isolated finding should not cause us to overestimate the importance of modeling.

Perhaps a more important reservation to the modeling hypothesis is this: If we say modeling is important, we have described a situation in which learning takes place, but we have said little about the nature of the learning strategies themselves. Given the importance of modeling, we do not know by what processes the child learns, or even how he selects models to imitate. We may find that models matter, but we must search for the child's major learning strategies in the acts he himself performs.

Self-motivated Practice

One of the most prominent acts the child performs while learning to communicate is practice. This is similar only in superficial form to such later forms as "practicing the piano." There is repetition of simple forms (similar to scales or elementary tunes), and there is concatenating of these forms into larger patterns. Such practice is different from piano practice in that no mother needs to force the child to practice. It is entirely self-motivated; the child seems simply to enjoy the esthetic experience of play with words.

Constant practice of musical patterns is, of course, the key to learning to play the piano. Is practice a major aspect of learning to communicate? It would strain credulity to argue that young children practice talking because they hope to be famous speakers in the sense that some children practice piano because they hope to be musicians when they grow up. Yet the practice itself could help communication whether the child knows it or not. One might even guess that the child's esthetic joy in making noise is nature's way of making him learn to talk.

Again, however, we must not assume that practice, just because it happens, represents an important learning strategy. There is evidence that learning can take place without it at some stages of development. As we discussed in Chapter 2, a baby whose throat operation prevented babbling for several months performed appropriately for his age on the day after his throat was repaired. The entire act of babbling, once thought important to sound development, is now considered to be of little importance. Children make sounds while babbling that they are unable to use in meaningful speech until many years later. Finally, there is the fact that children first learn to use irregular verbs correctly (run–ran), but later regularize them—in spite of having practiced the correct forms. In this case, practice seems unimportant; learning apparently results from inducing and applying rules, or what the learning theorist calls "generalization."

Rule-Induction

Brown and Bellugi (1964) speak of a syntax acquisition process, which they call *induction of latent structure*. This refers to a sequence in which a child hears a number of sentences that use similar syntactic constructions. Through his ability to generalize, the child comes implicitly to realize what rules are being followed. (A wide spectrum of evidence that such induction does occur is presented in the book you are reading.)

Our understanding of this induction process is very incomplete. Some researchers have guessed that such induction is simply stimulus-generalization learning cued by the order of words in sentences. This explanation is incomplete because word order by itself does not provide enough cues to deep structure. Yet the induction process certainly involves the child's making generalizations from limited sets of stimuli. Communication development, in fact, is characterized by generalizations made on the basis of extremely limited evidence. That is why language structure develops so fast. If the child waited for enough evidence to justify the generalizations he makes, he would never learn to talk.

A generalization made on insufficient evidence is bound to be an oversimplification—what we have called an overgeneralization. In Chapter 4, several examples of such overgeneralization were discussed. Regular tense endings on irregular verbs and regularized plural endings on nouns such as ox or sheep are among the many other instances that could be cited (see Ervin, 1964).

This evidence suggests the following rule-induction sequence:

1. The child discovers some meaning or concept or task that has communicative implications.
2. Closely related to this, the child discovers in his environment a new piece of the code that speakers in his language community use in apparent conjunction with this speech function.
3. The child overgeneralizes the function of the discovered piece of code—as does the scientist in the "implications" section of a research report—and applies it to a larger class of events. Given that there are fewer pieces in the child's code than kinds of speech events, many utterances that employ these overgeneralized rules will appear (to adults) to be rather "quaint errors"—just as many research reports written a generation ago now seem pleasantly naïve.
4. The child receives mixed reinforcement about his overgeneralized usage.
5. The child sorts out some events in which he has been using the rule with unhappy consequences. These he forms into a new class or classes, and searches the linguistic environment for a new general rule to cover the exceptional cases.
6. Discovering such a rule, the child again overgeneralizes it to some events for which it is inappropriate.

And it should be repeated that overgeneralization is the flip side of differentiation. Global overgeneralized categories are grist for differentiation and vice versa. (Readers familiar with Piaget's thought will note similarities with the concepts of assimilation and accommodation.)

The concept of rule induction raises as many questions as it resolves. We know very little about what particular events in the environment (home or school) will best facilitate rule induction. But some tactics are *not* likely to help much:

1. Teaching rules or principles explicitly in the absence of appropriate application to meaningful communication.
2. Imitating children exactly or forcing them to imitate you.
3. Correcting children's improper grammar, without understanding and attention to what the child is communicating.

As to what we *should* do, we must be more vague (but we shall elaborate some in the next chapter). Basically, we need to give children a chance to operate in circumstances in which communication can help them. Probably nothing is more helpful than a chance to operate within the most natural of all communication settings—conversation.

HUMPTY DUMPTY REASSEMBLED

Now for the impossible task of putting this together—or saying it all at once. This happens in Table 5. The learning strategies discussed in this chapter are listed on one axis, and the major aspects of development upon the other. An X at the intersection of a learning strategy and an aspect of development means that that strategy is important to that phase of communication development. A question mark (?) indicates that the learning strategy may be of importance; we are not certain at the present time.

Two things are immediately evident: (1) There are many question marks (because the research field is young and children are complex), and (2) most of the Xs are for the rule-induction learn-

table **5**

LEARNING STRATEGIES IN COMMUNICATION DEVELOPMENT

	ASPECTS OF DEVELOPMENT				
LEARNING PROCESSES	*Early Syntax*	*Later Syntax (Transformations & Exceptions)*	*Sounds*	*Meaning*	*Pragmatics (usage)*
Operant Conditioning		X		?	X
Imitation		?	X	X	
Modeling	?	?	?		
Practice			?		
Rule induction (overgeneralization)	X	?	X	X	X

X—important
?—may be of importance

ing process (which is, of course, the process about which we know least). Beyond this, we can make the following educated guesses.

Early syntax, which children are strongly biologically predisposed to acquire, is learned almost solely through rule-governed overgeneralization. This does not deny the fact that the environment is important here. A child must generalize on the basis of the language he hears. If that language is not correct standard American English, the child will obviously not learn correct standard American English. Beyond this, it is possible that syntax can be taught in some cases through modeling.

Later syntax (exceptions to general rules, and complex transformations) is learned very differently from early syntax. The process is much slower. The older child either is less of a linguistic genius than the young child (probable), or the problems he faces are more complex. As mentioned in Chapter 4, we know that certain rules are acquired late. But we know little about how these rules are learned. Due to the slowness of learning, the sort of powerful rule induction responsible for early syntax is unlikely. The best candidates for important places are imitation and modeling, in the context of operant conditioning.

The acquisition of *sounds* is also shrouded in mystery. Children certainly practice a great deal with sounds, but there is only very limited evidence that this is important to learning. Imitation likewise occurs and is probably important in working out some sound patterns. Obviously, a child must hear the sounds of a language to learn it, so in that broad sense, imitation is vital. But most important seems to be induction of rules from perceived speech. The ability to distinguish between sounds and to follow difficult rules about what sounds go where is about as remarkable and rapid as acquisition of syntax.

Even less is known about the acquisition of *meaning.* Clearly, much of what the child learns in this area is learned through imitation (using a particular label to refer to a particular thing). However, imitation alone cannot account for the child's ability to operate within the system of semantic markers and selection restrictions discussed in Chapter 5. Some rule-induction strategies may affect this learning; a kind of overgeneralization appears to take place in children's concept learning.

In the area of *pragmatics,* there is little evidence. We guess that learning in this area is about a half-and-half mix of operant conditioning (learning resulting from how people react to your communication), and rule induction. The rule induction can be seen to operate in the fact that we often know what is appropriate in a particular situation without even having encountered a similar situation. There is a sense in which patterns of usage, like rules of syntax, allow the speaker infinite numbers of alternatives out of which to create messages.

CONCLUDING APOLOGY

This model of how children learn to talk is like an egg reassembled—very fragile, with many cracks. We apologize, but we also feel that the perspective provided by this chapter can serve as a basis for some recommendations about how we can make things better. The rest of this book concentrates upon offering such advice.

Read This

BROWN, ROGER, and URSULA BELLUGI. "Three Processes in the Child's Acquisition of Syntax," *Harvard Educational Review* 34 (1964), 133–151; *also* in Eric Lenneberg (ed.), *New Directions in the Study of Language,* Cambridge, Mass.: MIT Press, 1965, *and* in Roger Brown, *Psycholinguistics,* New York: Free Press, 1970.

This article was one of the first attempts to talk in meaningful terms about the learning of grammar. Extremely well written.

ERVIN, SUSAN M. "Imitation and Structural Change in Children's Language," in Eric Lenneberg (ed.), *New Directions in the Study of Language.* Cambridge, Mass.: MIT Press, 1964.

Ervin discusses learning strategies and gives a large number of examples of overgeneralization in child speech.

chapter 9

TEACHING COMMUNICATION
TO CHILDREN

This chapter discusses problems in communication instruction
and proposes a strategy for improving speech skills. In the theoretical portion of the chapter, we consider some issues involved
in teaching grammar to children, both in traditional and "new
grammar" formats, and suggest that a teaching strategy based
upon functions of speaking is the best approach to communication instruction.

Sample procedures that can be used in the classroom also are
presented. We suggest only a few and describe them only in general terms because we have found that exercises and lessons borrowed from a book are usually less effective than those springing
from the teacher's personality and a set of principled goals.

TEACHING GRAMMAR

Recently, many theorists and researchers have argued that advances in psycholinguistics make it possible to teach children
grammar effectively. In our view, this argument is only half true.
It assumes more than we know and has some potentially dangerous consequences.

First, we should state the positive side. Research in developmental psycholinguistics has brought many ideas to the fore that
can be useful to elementary instruction. "Applied" psycholin-
guists usually have urged teachers to be more concerned with
knowledge learned by children and less concerned with surface

aspects of behavior on any given occasion. Teachers who follow this advice usually place less stress upon articulation errors, spelling, and the number of words in a child's vocabulary than do teachers unfamiliar with psycholinguistics. The change on the part of some teachers from articulation and vocabulary to emphasis on grammatical development is a healthy one. For example, a psycholinguistically oriented elementary teacher evaluating children participating in creative dramatics will probably pay less attention to gestures and expressions and greater attention to language structures.

These are some benefits of a teacher's knowing about developmental psycholinguistics. But the application of such principles suggests three interrelated problems:

> *Problem 1.* Developmental psycholinguistics as a research field is still in its infancy. Teachers must exercise great care in attempting classroom applications of still incomplete theories.
>
> *Problem 2.* Although research to date has given us some tools with which to evaluate children's grammatical development, almost nothing is known about trying to teach them grammar. Classroom attempts to teach grammar explicitly to young children (no matter how well intentioned) will probably fail. Further, these attempts may have dangerous side effects on the children and the general classroom atmosphere.
>
> *Problem 3.* Even if we could explicitly teach grammar to children, there is no evidence that it would significantly improve their communication skills. Because a major task of education is to improve communication abilities (speaking, reading, writing, listening), this reservation becomes important.

As these three problems indicate, teaching grammar rules to children does not necessarily help them communicate. Basically, the reason is this: When children come to school, they already know most of the grammar, but they only know it *implicitly*. This means that they speak grammatical sentences. But they may not even be able to define what sentences are. If you try to teach a child rules of grammar, you are not increasing what he knows. You are only increasing what he knows that he knows. And knowing what you know does not always cause better performance. Psychiatrists, for example, have studied the subconscious springs of behavior in great detail but this does not necessarily help them cope with their families and friends.

A simpler example relates to the same point. Give an eight-year-old child a bicycle and two hours to play with it. At the end of that time, he will be zooming up and down hills in wild, frightening abandon. At this point, call him aside and begin teaching him techniques to improve his skill. "Be sure to move your legs with fluid motion in an easy natural arc," you might say. "Grip the handlebars tightly, but hold your arms in a state of relaxed readiness. Head up! Eyes straight ahead." Ten minutes of such talk would probably suffice to make the child unable to ride or destroy his enthusiasm for it or both. Perhaps some kinds of knowledge are best left implicit.

This analogy may apply to attempts by some psycholinguistically oriented educators to teach grammar to children. Teaching grammar, particularly in secondary-school English class, has enjoyed a long tradition even though there has never been much evidence that students' speech or writing is improved by such instruction. Some educational theorists apparently believe that recent developments in linguistic theory now make teaching grammar practical. Linguists themselves do not argue this position. There is really no evidence to support it. Rather, the idea that "new linguistics" is more effectively teachable than "old linguistics" seems to be wishful thinking on the part of frustrated teachers—"If I teach them *new* grammar, they will *finally* learn to diagram sentences, and tell the difference between like and as!" This vision is not only misleading, but dangerous.

In the first place, it is dangerous because "new grammar" stands firmly against declaring one kind of sentence to be "proper grammar," and another frequently used sentence ("Winston tastes good *like* a cigarette should") to be bad grammar. New grammar is only descriptive, and according to new grammar, "like" is as grammatical as "as" because speakers use it.

In the second place, not only is using old methods to teach new grammar sure to fail, but also the act of making such an attempt can poison the classroom atmosphere. At best, children will see prescribed structures as schoolroom "trivia-academic games," which are important only in class and on tests. If this happens, the "learned" structures will not be used in everyday speech, and the schoolroom will become (justifiably) an object of student ridicule. But this is not the *worst* thing that is likely to happen. If the teacher is particularly forceful or authoritarian in teaching grammar (even new grammar), he may ruin the entire classroom atmosphere in the attempt. High-powered, high-content teaching in instances where failure is likely makes learning unlikely, a fact pointed out forcefully by John Holt in *How Children Learn* and by Charles Silberman in *Crisis in the Classroom*.

There is one final problem with emphasizing grammar in communication instruction. Linguistics deals with no unit larger than the sentence. Knowing grammar is of little help in putting complex ideas together, constructing rhetorical strategies, or reading an entire page for overall comprehension.

All these problems make the teaching of grammar very difficult. But we are still left with the issue: Given that we want children to communicate effectively, what kind of teaching strategies do we employ toward that end? The answer, we suggest, is to utilize teaching strategies based upon pragmatic aspects of speech development (that aspect of development discussed in Chapter 6). The following sections will show the benefits of such an approach and sketch some sample teaching strategies.

FORM AND FUNCTION IN INSTRUCTIONAL STRATEGIES

If it is unwise to teach grammar directly, how can educators aid grammar learning? To answer this question, it is necessary to pose another: How is it that the child (who knows most of the grammar before school) goes about acquiring a new grammatical rule? McNeill (1966, p. 64) states that a child ordinarily learns a new distinction of adult grammar not because he is taught it by some adult or peer, but because the child himself discovers a new "meaning for which he must find some means of differentiation and expression." In this view, the child is innately structured so that the acquisition of grammatical principles is an easy task, provided he has some use for them.

As we discussed in some detail in Chapter 8, what seems to

happen is this: First, the child learns some new function language can perform—to get the milk passed from the other end of the table or to get his parents to allow him to stay up late. Next, the language learner searches the language behavior in his environment until he locates the grammar rule or rules needed to express this new distinction in meaning. Mastery of that rule and incorporation of the rule into his usage follow quickly because the child's innate linguistic endowment makes this easy.

It is not the mastery of the new grammar rules themselves that holds the key to the development of new structures, but rather *the connecting of these rules with real-life speech situations*. If this is so, then the best way to teach grammar is to teach pragmatics. Thus teachers can relieve frustrations over "bad grammar" while teaching something more palatable. As medieval explorers discovered, it is sometimes easiest to get East by sailing West. If we base our communication teaching upon functions of speaking, grammar will be learned—perhaps not in time for the first six-weeks test, but eventually.

This does not mean to imply that function can be taught with no reference to the state of the child's grammatical development. There are some grammatical distinctions that no child learns until age eight or nine, and trying to teach him the accompanying functions is likely to be futile. Educators need to study in detail each pupil's performance in grammar and function, and design appropriate teaching strategies on the basis of that information.

Further, it should be clear by now that form and function in speaking are highly interdependent. On any given occasion, a teacher may have to assist one of these aspects of development or the other. Our advice that elementary instructions focus upon function is a pragmatic hypothesis based upon what we know about children, *but it is not an absolute rule*. There are occasions in which a schoolchild needs small amounts of help with grammar structure. The teacher certainly should provide it.

In addition to teaching function to aid learning of grammatical form, educators should help children learn rules of pragmatics. It is important that children know rules of appropriate usage in varieties of speech situations. We never put people in asylums for bad grammar, but we routinely commit those who lose the ability to keep straight the rules of usage—who fly into a rage for no reason or laugh in church. A thorough knowledge of verbal behaviors appropriate in varied situations is essential to survival in a complex world.

Finally, whether teachers are teaching grammar or function, they *should not teach rules explicitly,* apart from situations in which they are appropriate. The specialized terminology used in this book and in research should not filter down into the classroom. Teachers should know and keep in mind the aspects of situational context discussed in Chapter 7, but should not force children to memorize jargon they will have little use for unless they become teachers themselves. Rather, teachers should formulate classroom activities that will help the children develop implicit knowledge about how speech varies according to context. The children can learn the jargon when they go to college and read this book. This does not necessarily mean that children should never be taught the rules or principles which govern language. It may, on occasion, be helpful for a child to be able to verbalize a principle he is using. The point here is that the child will not be able to use a rule just because he has memorized it.

SOME SAMPLE COMMUNICATION-TEACHING STRATEGIES

Now comes the part when we tell you what to do in that classroom full of real-life children. More specifically, we list some general alternatives you should consider when planning units of instruction. Before you read the suggestions, read this warning:

Caution: The literal translation of these exercises into instructional strategies may be hazardous to learning!

This warning is necessary for at least two reasons. First, these ideas appear here as logical extensions of our theory of communicative development. None of them has received careful experimental testing; several have never even been tried in school settings. Second, a warning is necessary because these exercises are outgrowths of *our* teaching personalities. Each teacher must formulate his own set of procedures based upon his teaching style.

With these cautions, let us proceed to concrete suggestions. Because the main thrust of our recommendations centers around a function-based approach to communication instruction, our first (and most detailed) suggestions focus upon this area. Following this are some suggestions about other areas of instruction, and about the classroom environment as a whole.

In Chapter 7, we discussed in some detail five aspects of situations that have important effects on communication. For simplicity, we lump our suggestions here into those same five categories. It is probably worthwhile to restate the fact that these five variables all interact with each other. We list exercises under individual categories so that you can gain a balanced approach by giving some emphasis to each area.

Throughout all these suggestions, a dominant theme is that a teacher's strongest teaching lever is *modeling*—being an example of how he wants students to act. Mostly, this means that teachers must constantly monitor the classroom situation and adjust their behavior to changing communication climates. So often, many of us have been intent upon "getting the message across" and "covering the material," and have adjusted poorly to the situation.

A. *Personal Context.* How communication is affected by the specific people who are communicating. Suggestions:

1. Students practice in "audience analysis." Run off on ditto or write on the blackboard some brief messages. (Keep them interesting to students—don't ask a first grader to argue international politics.) Students discuss how they would present this message to varied audiences. Alternatively, students could prepare speeches, make posters, break into groups and prepare persuasive campaigns for each of the different audiences. This works best when the message can really be presented by children to some of the audiences. Such instant effectiveness feedback teaches well. Finally, such exercises should be accompanied by literal sprinklings of discussions of tactics employed, effectiveness, possible side effects, and so forth.

2. Communication with unusual people. This odd subtitle refers to placing children in real-life encounters that necessitate wide shifts in communication behavior. This can be

accomplished during field trips, if children are encouraged to talk with guides, policemen, and children enrolled in schools for the blind or retarded. Trips to various places of business offer chances to talk to people who are extremely formal (in a department store or high-priced shoe store), or less formal (in a neighborhood delicatessen or ice cream parlor). Little or no instruction is usually needed. Activities that point out how language behavior varies according to the people present can be fruitful—not to point out "principles," but to facilitate future adaptations.

3. Role-playing or dramatics. This can be effective either structured or unstructured—with story lines or open-ended. The important item here is to change the nature of the situation by entering and exiting characters—showing how behavior varies according to communication. With younger, more self-conscious children, many of the same functions can be accomplished through the use of puppets.

4. Telephoning. Split children into "teams" of two, and have them pretend to talk to each other by telephone. Then instruct one of the team to be a "parent," and talk to the other. Then switch. Then have both be parents. Other possibilities: storekeepers, businessmen, teachers, preachers, the President.

5. Teacher as model. Keep tuned to how the composition of classes or discussion groups varies with absences or new faces. Such changes can also be grist for discussion. After the principal visits and sits in the back of the room for a half hour, start a discussion of how you and the children behaved differently.

B. *Conversational Context.* How communication is affected by what is said before and by what is likely to be said next. Suggestions:

1. "Out of context" game. Orally or in writing, expose students to one message, then a short summary or quotes from the first message. Discuss ways the summary or quote is accurate or inaccurate in terms of the first passage. Does it convey the whole meaning of the first passage or only part? If you (student) wrote the first passage and somebody else summar-

ized you with the second passage, how would you feel—happy, angry, amused, sad? Why?

2. Passages with gaps. This works much like the out of context game. Students are presented with incomplete stories, descriptions, or other passages. The beginning, middle, or end could be omitted. Students compose their own version of missing section, and alternative adaptations to the situation form the basis for student discussions. Both these procedures would lend themselves to mimeographed "workbooks" for older children.

3. Incomplete dramas or puppet shows. Give children partial stories or plays. Let them act out their own endings. A variation: Give the initial situation and a required ending and let students construct the show which gets to that ending. Groups of students (three to five in a group) could discuss in advance how to do the shows—amount of planning could be varied from much to none. And, of course, either groups or the entire class can discuss the success of attempts afterward.

4. Be a model. When a student makes a remark that is *clearly* inappropriate to what was said before and the general drift of discussion, the teacher might inform him (nonhumiliatingly) of the inappropriateness. When you want to change discussion topics but the class is still interested in what you wish to change from, be subtle; shift topics by steering conversation gently. Make your remarks appropriate to what has been said, and connect what has been said to what you want to discuss next.

C. *Content Context.* How communication is affected by the topic under discussion and student interest in that topic. Suggestions:

There is, of course, little need to teach children to be interested in something—children usually turn their natural curiosity in some direction. And there probably is little chance that a student can be taught to appreciate everything that captures the fancy of his teacher. What children need if they are to develop this aspect of their communication skills is *room to operate*—to do things that matter without too much interference. The best way to provide this is to allow children to choose a project of their own. Teachers should, of course, aid in project selection to avoid caprice and boondoggling. But once the project area and objectives have been worked out, children should be given free rein to experiment and innovate. Teachers can guide and listen critically and sometimes make procedural suggestions. But avoid steering conversations around to old "educational tritisms" to "help the children learn." These projects are not recess or "enrichment exercises," they are the heart of a student-centered communication curriculum. A final caution: Make initial projects small and allow children time to work out their self-motivated learning procedures. The first few attempts are likely to be confusing, but later students move with surprising speed. The suggestions that follow can all be used by individual students or by discussion groups. Particularly with younger children, group projects probably should be used more often.

1. Writing shows or plays. Children can and will do surprising things with this activity if teachers do not make the act of composition formidable with excessive warnings and frequent corrections of details of grammar and style. This can also be done in groups, provided all group members have some interest in the subject. Finally, small projects should be completed before more complex ones are attempted.

2. Pursue interests or hobbies. Such projects as growing plants, keeping pets, and doing small experiments in physics or chemistry can provide a framework for activity. Here the teacher treads a fine line between things that can be done in school (growing plants, experiments, etc.) and other activities too grandiose for the classroom (raising pets or produce, sending up weather balloons). In many cases, however, this dilemma can be solved by doing many activities outside the schoolroom during class hours. Four walls do not an education make. And it should be restated that this is not "enrichment crafts hour," but a vital part of your communication curriculum. A child is better off talking, reading, and writing about a cow than being sullen during a chemistry lesson.

3. Act on problems. This is a group activity of tremendous potential. Within the school, neighborhood, and city there are

dozens of problems that catch the students' fancy and capture their concern: petty theft, littering, abuse of a vacant lot, pollution from a nearby plant. Students should be encouraged (mainly in groups) to tackle these problems, to plot persuasive strategies, attempt fund raising, and generally try to make things better. The fact that he helped get new linoleum in the cafeteria may be a child's greatest source of pride from his school year. Consider the gold mine of communication practice in writing leaflets, business letters, or letters of outrage, or telephoning a radio station to ask for time on the air—let alone writing and executing a script to fill the time.

4. Be a model. Allow yourself your own interests, of course, but be genuinely open and probing as you try to help students to communicate about their interests. And when the class seems very interested in discussing a topic that is not what you wanted to "cover" that day, you should consider being flexible—and covering your material later. This is an invitation not to be wishy-washy, but simply to be open, willing to learn, and stronger than those who only know how to ask one set of questions.

D. *Task Context.* How communication is affected by the goals communicators are trying to accomplish. Suggestions:

1. Grammar games. Play games in which children are put in verbal situations that require responses using specific grammatical structures. For young children, this can be quite simple—for example, a question starting with "why" requires in answer a clause using "because." Other ideas include: (a) Having one child say a simple sentence and subsequent players add a thought to it while still using only one sentence, and (b) having children "play" with complex embedding structures by expanding fun sentences (see Moffett, 1968). Such games also could be used to teach situational demands of function.

2. Question asking. This is one function of language that education must develop. Children naturally ask questions; teachers should help them develop their questioning ability into a sensitive probing instrument. Games such as "20 questions" that systematically attack and solve problems of identification can be helpful in this regard. Without ever using for-

midable words such as "scientific method" children can be taught how to ask questions of data and obtain their own answers. All these sorts of procedures can be undertaken by students in pairs and small groups, and the teacher needs only to consult with those having trouble. If this results in a classroom atmosphere that is loud and chaotic, do not be shocked; children can work very well in such an atmosphere with some supervision and some inviting learning tasks. One final suggestion: Play with riddles and encourage your children to bring new ones to school.

3. Rhythm and rhyme games. A favorite nursery-school game is to give children a pair of long sticks, which they bang together in time to music. This might have some useful carry-overs to elementary school with more complex rhythms and perhaps use with spoken language as well as with songs. The rhythm of a ballad, for example, could provide interesting vocal and rhythm games. Allow children to make up rhythms of their own and then invite them (and aid them when necessary) to set the rhythms to words. Rhyme games can be an equally rich source for games: "Make a word that rhymes with ———." Or have one child say a word and each child around a circle tries to rhyme it. Or have a pair of children take turns saying words and rhyming words said by the partner.

4. Verbal mediation. Sometimes both language and ability to do something can be aided if we talk about what we are doing as we do it. Sometimes practice in such verbal mediation can give us added problem-solving ability. One way to practice this would be to talk (to yourself or others) about a picture as you draw it. Another would be to manipulate puppets and describe what each is doing. Verbal mediation can also be used when a child has difficulty with a task. The teacher can encourage him to verbalize his reasoning (talk his way through it). Such a procedure often leads to self-correction because the student hears what he is doing wrong as he says it. This procedure also helps the teacher pinpoint the source of the child's problem. Eventually, the child will learn to talk his way through problems with no outside assistance.

Mastery of such critical "dialogue-with-self" strategies can
be a tremendous help to learning ability.

5. Model. The main function of teacher-as-model with
these ideas is to exhibit an enthusiasm for the esthetics of
language use—a sense of joy about the way the parts of the
code fit together and provide almost endless play opportunities. It is only when children see language used as a dry academic activity that games such as those described above will
seem "silly" to them.

E. *Surrounding physical context*. How communication is affected by the place in which you are communicating and visual
cues to sentence meanings. Suggestions:

1. Context-conflict games. The experimental finding that
asking a question about one item (say, a glass) while holding
before a child a picture of a different item (a spoon) causes
confusion leads to several game possibilities. If not tied to deep
feelings of failure–fear, a game in which pictures are used to
trip up answerers could be fun. It could also provide evidence
that visual communication cues are less dependable than linguistic ones.

2. Context as aid. This is the more constructive side of the
same coin. Here, use of pictures, dolls, or even little role-plays
could aid children in understanding structures that are difficult for them. Such cues could be used to help students see that
in sentences like

"The elephant is kissed by the bear."

it is the bear who kisses. After practice with the context items
has made children more aware of the linguistic structures,
they may be able to interpret them better. But we must be
careful not to ask here what Piaget calls "the American question": "Can we make them do it *younger?*" Techniques such
as these will probably be helpful if the child is "ready" to
learn a distinction. If he is not, they will probably make little
difference.

3. Role-plays with varied scenes. Have children construct
stories or act out plays based on being in exotic and ordinary
places. Discussions could bring out the importance of scene to

communication. Some sample places: a country store, a department store, a gas station, at home alone, in church, in a haunted house, in an old castle, in a crowded modern skyscraper, in a barnyard.

GENERAL RECOMMENDATIONS

Aside from these fairly specific suggestions for a function-based communication curriculum, we have a few more general pieces of advice for teachers particularly interested in communication.

First, start simple and move later to complex ideas. With young children especially, do not attempt to move too fast. Rather, let children generate their own enthusiasm—and let that set the pace. With young children you will also desire to emphasize manipulation of objects, rhythm play, and overcoming "stage fright" and shyness—and fear of failure. Using puppets and having children talk through them often helps in this regard, as does breaking the class into groups of three or four, so there are few listeners.

As children grow up, they still manipulate things, but the nature of the manipulation changes from physical (hitting sticks together) to cognitive (how can we best make this plant grow?). Continued opportunities to make such manipulations and see the results—and compare results with predictions—are valuable scientific and linguistic training because they provide a need for structures—for example, "If I do A then I would expect B to happen."

It can be seen from the suggestions to this point that our theories are not actualized in any set of preplanned textbooks or prewritten lesson plans. We do not think they ever will be, for what we are asking is that each teacher plan his communication curriculum on the basis of where the students are and what they need to learn.

Classroom atmosphere should not be preplanned, but rather should be spontaneous and exciting, even if occasionally chaotic. The students should be accustomed to working individually, in groups of two to three or five to six, and as an entire class. Much of the teacher's work should be oriented toward solving individual problems and making students more able to learn from each other. The teacher should be more of a consultant and decision maker—and less of an information machine. It should be evident by now that we advocate a communication atmosphere very different from what exists in most elementary classrooms. We despair at too much quiet in elementary schools. The giant of child psychology, Jean Piaget, has often observed that children need to accompany actions and thinking with talking. Such talking is natural and aids learning. Just as talking is an important aid to thinking, frequent open-ended discussions provide opportunities for students to test and sharpen their ideas and perceptions against those of other children. Further, the activity of criticizing others' ideas and giving reasons for the reactions exercises a child's thinking and provides him with dialogue practice.

Within all this, every class should contain, so far as possible, a heterogeneous mix of students. Varieties of speakers provide the best possible laboratory for increasing speech and comprehension. Not only should classes be integrated in terms of sex, ethnicity, and social class according to the full spirit of the law, but also there should be more mixing of children of varying intelligence. Even age segregation is in some ways detrimental to learning: Children should have ample communication opportunities with people of all ages. This wide range of students is helpful in many ways. First, it teaches that there are many kinds of communication strategies, each appropriate in some kinds of communication situations. In addition to ethnic differences, temperamental differences would be more evident. Some children are loud and aggressive, others are quiet and reserved. In a heterogeneous classroom, the student sees all these communication strategies at work. He is then free to choose varying models for varying situations. Second, such a classroom provides practice in audience analysis. The child will learn that it is unproductive to speak the same way all the time. In short, a mixed classroom is a generalized aid to learning patterns of usage.

Finally, development of communication skill comes not through memorization of principles of *any* aspect of communication. Rather, it emerges through using (exercising) the communicating "muscles" in encounters with important problems. We argued in detail against teaching principles of grammar. We would argue equally strongly against teaching principles of rhetoric, usage, extralinguistic expression, or reading. *Children learn to communicate by communicating.* Only *after* a child has learned what to do will the statement of a principle be of use to him. To foster such learning, children must communicate more than they usually do in today's classrooms. Emphases upon orderly calm and "keeping quiet" have to go. These must be replaced by discussion as an everyday educational staple. Communicating is the curriculum, not enrichment. Do not introduce a topic for discussion with, "Well, let's have a discussion about snow." In addition to being boring, this procedure sets no goals worth obtaining. The result will be a lot of talk going no place. What we should do instead is set goals in cooperation with students and let the students attain them through discussion. Emphasis then is on the discussion not as a phase of school, but as a tool for getting things done.

And remember that it is possible to have discussions without teaching a set of rules first. If you are worried that without teaching rules you will have nothing to test over, eliminate your tests. They do not help learning, yet there is a steady diet of them at each stage of education. Psychologists would say that such a constant unpleasant stimulus would cause unpleasant associations with the rest of learning even if the rest were fun. And the rest is not always fun—although it usually could be. Who ever said learning *had* to be dull?

Read This

MAY, FRANK. *Teaching Language as Communication to Children.* Columbus, Ohio: Merrill, 1967.
This book reviews research evidence concerning teaching communication to children in a coherent and readable fashion. It suggests what communication skills must be taught and some ways to teach them.
MOFFETT, JAMES. *Teaching the Universe of Discourse.* New York: Houghton Mifflin, 1968.

Moffett outlines a comprehensive theory for teaching children to communicate using writing, speaking, reading, and drama. He shares our bias against teaching grammar, and his case in this area is worth reading. His student-centered approach to almost everything is healthy and inventive.

POSTMAN, NEIL, and CHARLES WEINGARTNER. *Teaching as a Subversive Activity*. New York: Delacorte, 1969.

This book should hearten any teacher who has run into disheartening experiences trying to make constructive changes in clasroom procedures. With an emphasis on teaching communication, these authors cut through much educational baloney.

chapter 10

SCHOOL, COMMUNICATION, AND MINORITY-GROUP CHILDREN

It is fashionable for books concerned with education and language to mention special problems of minority-group children. Such mention is usually stuck in the last few pages of the book, as were 1940 Negroes on a Greyhound bus. We follow this fashion only because our discussion of the communicative skills of disadvantaged children rests upon our entire framework of thought and thus is most understandable at this point.

As government social engineering mixes more children of varying ethnic backgrounds, more teachers are exposed to "special problems of disadvantaged students." The "problem" is that children from minority groups usually speak "nonstandard" dialects of English. This means that there is some consistent and recognizable way in which their speech is different from the speech of middle-class whites from Peoria, Illinois. Many educators feel that this nonstandard speaking accounts for the fact that minority-group children do poorly in school.

NONSTANDARD DIALECTS

The use of the term "nonstandard" obviously implies the existence of a standard. Before we can talk about nonstandard dialects, it makes sense to ask about the standard dialect. In this country, the use of the term "standard English" has generally been confined to English teachers and their friends. It is used to mean "proper" or "correct" English. Standard English is the form of speech described in old-fashioned grammar books. As such, it is actually spoken by few people. However, it is a form of speech usually *expected* from well-educated people. Fortunately or unfortunately, it has come to be identified as the speech of educated, white, middle-class Americans. It is important to remember that even when educated, white, middle-class Americans talk, they often use incomplete sentences, which are not strictly grammatical. There is nothing wrong with this. It's just a fact of communication. No one is likely to remark about it, unless the speaker's way of talking can be identified as a *dialect* of English. The difference between the everyday mistakes one is likely to make and a dialect variation is that ordinary errors are likely to be random and inconsistent, whereas a dialect is comprised of consistent and predictable variations from standard English. Sometimes we might say: "These boys were playing," and sometimes: "These boys was playing." Such departures from the rules of standard English cannot be predicted. In a dialect, however, the specific variations from the standard form are quite recognizable and predictable. That is why comedians and actors are able to sound like hillbillies or Jewish mothers—they can identify the consistent differences between the speech of these groups and the speech of the typical middle-class, white American. All the skillful actor needs to do is imitate the major characteristics of some dialect, and he will be identified as a member of the group with which that dialect is associated.

This leads to another characteristic of a dialect: It is usually associated with a particular group of people, who have in common something besides the way they talk. Dialects are most often associated with geographical areas; so we have a southern dialect, shared by people who live in the South and southeastern parts of the country. It cuts across politics; you hear it in George Wallace as well as William Fulbright. To a certain extent, it also cuts across social class boundaries. The "rednecks" and the country club set in any southern town will sound alike in many respects. Dialects are also associated with second-language learning. People who do not have English as their native language will tend to sound different from native speakers when they learn English. The Puerto Ricans in New York City and the Mexican-

Americans in the southwest are typical of groups that speak foreign-language influenced dialects.

People who talk about the problem of nonstandard dialects in the schools are most likely to be talking about the speech of the black child in the inner-city schools of our large northern cities. It is perhaps cynical, but in many ways true, to say that the predominantly white middle-class educational establishment in these cities has, in the past ten years or so, been confronted with large numbers of children who do not sound like white middle-class children sound, and this has caused a problem. The question is, whose problem is it? And what is to be done about it?

Much research and thought during past years has focused around this question. Early researchers believed that black speech simply represented a disorganized and poorly articulated version of white speech. These researchers concluded that nonstandard speakers were deficient in grammar. This position is known as the *deficit* theory.

Most preschool intervention programs in the 1960s were based upon the deficit hypothesis. Educators felt that if minority children could be taught standard English, their school achievement problems would vanish. This was an attractive theory because it attributed a whole host of failure problems to one observable cause—inferior language. However, later research demonstrated that nonstandard varieties of English are not inferior. Recent scholarship has pointed out that black nonstandard English is as highly structured and rule-governed as standard English.

It is now more fashionable in scholarly circles to say that dialects of English are simply different from each other. According to this *difference* theory of American dialects, no dialect is inferior to others. Educational problems result not because minority children know no grammar, but because the school atmosphere offers instruction only in an alien grammar. The solution of difference theorists is *bidialectal instruction*—teaching children grammar of both their native dialect and standard English in the early grades. In theory, children will be fluent in both dialects and able to use each when it is most appropriate.

The difference approach (bidialectal instruction) seems preferable to the deficit approach, but in actual practice the differences between the two approaches may be quite slight. Minority children are still required to learn society's predominant dialect—a dialect spoken by people with whom they are rarely allowed to associate. Teachers still feel that the dominant dialect is "standard" and that instruction in nonstandard dialects is to be tolerated only as a lever to promote learning of the standard. Because there is still little "good literature" written in nonstandard dialects, the older student only has standard English books to read. So the child is, in effect, asked to enter a new speech community in which he is a second-class citizen.

The inadequacies of programs based upon difference theory lead us to ask: Are the grammar differences between these two dialects important and pervasive enough to cause such difficulty? The answer seems to be "No, not really that important." If we examine black English, for example, we find that dialect to differ from standard English only by a few grammatical rules and some pronunciation differences. The few differences in syntax occur mostly in surface structure. Differences in deep structure seem small indeed (Labov, 1970b).

The major differences between black English and standard English are summarized below.

SYNTACTIC FEATURES
1. The expression of possession is different. Standard English: "Joe's pencil"; nonstandard dialect: "Joe pencil."
2. Negation is expressed by double negatives or "ain't." Standard English: "I don't have a pencil"; dialect: "I ain't got no pencil."
3. Subject-verb agreement differs. Standard English: "We were there" or "They are here"; dialect: "We was there" or "They is here."
4. "S" is omitted from third-person singular verbs in the dialect. "He sings" becomes "He sing."
5. The use of "is" is not necessary in present-tense sentences. "I am going" or "He is here" become "I going" or "He here."
6. "If" constructions are changed. "I'll ask Mary if she wants to go" may be changed to "I'll ask Mary do she want to go."
7. The "ed" on past tense verbs may be omitted. "He walked" may become "He walk." (Note: Irregular past tense will not

be omitted. "Sang," will not become "sing," and "went" will not become "go.")

8. Future tense of verbs may be expressed differently. "I'm going to go" will be "I'm 'a go." "He's going to go" will be "He 'gon go."
9. "Be" may be used to express habitual action. "He be sick" means "He's always sick" as opposed to "He sick" meaning "He's sick right now."
10. Pronominal apposition will appear in the subject of a sentence. "John is funny" will be "John he funny." "Mary said to come in" will be "Mary she say to come in."

PHONOLOGICAL FEATURES

1. "R" may be omitted before consonants or if it is the last sound in a word. "Guard" will sound like "god," "carrot" will sound like "cat."
2. "L" may be omitted before consonants or if it is a final sound. "Help" will be "hep," "bowl" will be "bow."
3. Consonant clusters at the end of words will be shortened. "First" will be "firs," "told" will be "tol," "let's" will be "les."
4. Final consonants will be weaker. "Want" will sound like "wan."

Several things should be pointed out about this list of characteristics. First, it is not likely that any individual black child has in his speech all of these features. This list is a general description of features in the speech of a large group, and each individual has his own variation. Just as all speakers of standard English do not sound alike, so all speakers of the dialect do not sound alike. Additionally, the use of the dialect may vary according to the degree of formality in the situation, with fewer dialect features being found in very formal situations, and more being found in informal situations.

The second thing to remember about this list is that even if one found a child whose speech contained every feature listed, there is no reason to assume that his speech would be unintelligible to a listener. There is no real sacrifice of semantic information in the dialect, particularly when the speech is taken in context. The claim of many teachers that they cannot understand what the inner-city black child is saying may be due to something other than the child's speech. And there is certainly no evidence to suggest that because he speaks a nonstandard dialect, a black child cannot understand standard English.

Some people have suggested, in line with the deficient language point of view, that because the black child brought up in a poverty-stricken environment does not receive sufficient language stimulation in the home, he starts school with inadequately developed language skills. These people like to say that such children need language enrichment programs. Let us examine this view carefully. First, as we have pointed out at several points in this book, we do not know how much or what kind of language a child has to hear to learn how to talk. All we know is that he must be exposed to some language. So it is difficult to determine what constitutes "inadequate" language stimulation. Second, we have no evidence that inner-city black children fail to develop language. Indeed, the evidence is all to the contrary. On the playground or in the street they are just as talkative as any other children anywhere. This may not be true in the classroom, but that can (and should) be explained in other ways. The truth of the matter is that children learn to speak the language of their environment. If their parents and friends speak French, they learn French. And if their parents and friends speak a nonstandard dialect, they learn the dialect. They do not learn standard English. This is not the same thing as saying that their language development is inadequate.

FUNCTIONAL ASPECTS OF NONSTANDARD DIALECT

The question then becomes: If there are no significant syntactic or phonological differences between the nonstandard dialect of the black child and the standard English of the white teacher, where is the problem? It does appear that the economically handicapped black child is at a true disadvantage in our schools. But perhaps the problem is not a linguistic one, due to rules in the child's grammar, as much as a communicative one, due to attitudes about and uses of language.

As mentioned in Chapter 6, a child acquiring language is

learning much more than the rules of a grammar. He is also learning appropriate ways of using language in communication situations. One way in which cultures may be expected to differ from one another is in the kinds of communication situations they admit and in the rules for appropriate usage within these situations. Given that the typical disadvantaged black child and the typical middle-class white child are growing up and learning language in different cultures, it seems reasonable to expect that these two groups of children would be different in the ways they use language to communicate.

The differences in language usage between these two groups can perhaps best be seen by looking at an example of language use by a lower-status black child. The example given here is part of a conversation between a ten-year-old girl (G) and an older woman (W).* Both are black residents of Washington, D.C. G is describing a movie she saw.

> W: "Our Man Flint." Tell me about it, what was it about?
> G: It was zis strong. I' was about dis strong man. An' he was cu'.
> W: An' he was what?
> G: An he was cu'.
> W: Uh huh
> G: An' he dived off o' dat big thing, an' dived into de water.
> W: Dived off what big thing?
> G: I' was bou', i' was dese mount'ns.
> W: Okay. Go ahead. About the big man an' what?
> G: He see, he puts, he say, an he puts some o' dese girls in dese cans an' trow 'em.
> W: In cans?
> G: Un huh. An' put 'em in ne water.
> W: What for?
> G: For, for he c'n, for dey c'n go to de boa' an' be safe. For da thing.
> W: Well was he a good man or a bad man?
> G: He was a goo' man.
> W: Wha' was his name?
> G: FLIN'.
> W: Oh, that's right, okay, so go ahead, an' what happens?
> G: An', an' he ain', an' no more water wasn' comin' down. So he

* Reprinted from Bengt Loman, *Conversations in a Negro Dialect,* Washington, D.C.: Center For Applied Linguistics, pp. 155–158.

> dived off o' dat big mount'n an' dived into de water an' star'
> swimmin' over to da boa'.
> W: An' then what happened to the girls in . . .
> G: An' den', an', an', girls in ne can. Dey were, dey, de, de cans.
> Made 'em go to de boa', an' den ney take de girls out de can,
> an' put 'em in ne boa', 'n give 'em a towel an' wrap aroun' em.
> W: An' so then what happened?
> G: An nen na' was de e'. (the end)
> W: So then the girls were saved?
> G: Uh huh
> W: . . . So the whole movie was about Flint's saving these girls?
> G: Uh uh
> W: Well den what?
> G: I' was abou' our man Flin', an' nere was dis telephone, say
> boom, boom, boom, boom.
> W: Telephone, what did the telephone have to do with i'?
> G: I' was dis man.
> W: Uh huh
> G: An' he had some o' dese suggestures for Flin', some o' dese
> tricks for Flin', an' Flin' say he didn' need i'.
> W: Bu' wha' was zis man gonna do for Flin'?
> G: Nofin. See dis, dis world' wan'ed, destroy. Da' worl'. De other worl'

The first thing to notice about this interchange is the difficulty
W has in getting G to tell what the movie was about. W is asking for an overall summary statement, such as "Well, it was
about a plot to take over the world by people from outer space,
and Flint has to stop them by blowing up their space ship." Instead, G keeps giving descriptions of isolated instances, of things
that happened in the movie, rather than what the movie was
about. This tendency on the part of lower-status or disadvantaged children has been noted in their discussions of television
programs as well (Williams, 1970). The point is not that there is
anything wrong about describing particular instances of action in
the movie. The difficulty is that W, and the reader, have no context to relate these descriptions to. They become very difficult to
understand, as can be seen by W's questions. G seems to be assuming that W knows everything about the movie that she
knows, so that remarks like "an' he dived off o' dat big thing"
will be perfectly clear. W, of course, does not share the context.
She has not seen the movie, so she has to ask: "What big thing?"

This assumption of shared context where there is, in fact, no sharing, is a major characteristic of the speech of disadvantaged children, whether black or white.

One explanation for this is that the disadvantaged child is brought up in an environment where shared context is the usual thing. The child seldom has to speak with "outsiders," who have had different experiences and different points of view. His world is, in this sense, a narrow and close-knit one. The middle-class child, however, has encountered a broader range of communicative situations. Because he has more individual experiences that do not include everyone he knows, he is accustomed to having to explain things to people who were not present when things happened.

That is, because of environmental differences, the disadvantaged child is accustomed to using language differently from the middle-class child. This difference becomes particularly striking when the disadvantaged child begins school and encounters that very important outsider, the teacher, who does not share his experiences, his point of view. This probably marks the onset of his educational disadvantage.

A second characteristic of the speech of the typical disadvantaged child is a lack of *elaboration*. An elaborated sentence is one that puts two or three ideas (each of which could be a simple sentence) into one sentence, such as the sentence you are now reading. That sentence puts all these simple sentence ideas together:

1. Elaborated sentences combine ideas.
2. Each idea could be a simple sentence.
3. This sentence is elaborated.

The elaborated sentence we used to express all this is the kind of sentence middle-class children learn to speak. Elaborated sentences use large numbers of adjectives, dependent noun phrases and clauses, and complex embedded structures.

So middle-class American children use more elaborated sentences than lower-class children. This is a mixed blessing. Elaborated sentences can aid precision in some situations, but in other situations they can get in the way of communication. Like those high-suds detergents so popular in the 1950s, elaborated sentences can clog up interaction. As any political press conference will show, erudite, educated American English speakers can often use lots of words to say very little.

Even this often-cited difference between lower-class and middle-class speakers may not be as widespread as it appears to be. Williams and Naremore (1970), analyzing interactions of middle-class and lower-class children with adults, discovered that lower-class children are capable of using elaborated speech when called on to do so. The difference between the two groups of children seems to be that middle-class children use elaborated speech even when they don't have to.

If you want to see how this works, ask a four- or five-year-old middle-class child: "What games did you play today?" His response, if he feels comfortable around you, will be something like: "I played baseball with Jimmy and Karen and . . . um . . . we played in the street, and . . . um . . . we played until Eddie got hurt, . . . um . . . he fell down, . . . um . . . and then I had to go home for dinner." At each of these pauses the child will struggle to find something else to say and use the vocalized pause to "keep the floor" because he isn't finished elaborating. This child, because he has always been encouraged to talk a lot, *has come to love elaboration for its own sake*. A lower-class child, asked the same question, may answer it in a word or two. His answer is more precise, but to a teacher looking for elaboration, such a child may appear sullen or hostile.

By any measure, nonstandard usage is unacceptable to school teachers. Labov (1968) says that one reason for this is that many school teachers grew up in nonstandard-English neighborhoods and succeeded in school only by learning standard. This makes them more intolerant of nonstandard usage than most middle-class speakers.

So far our discussion has suggested that the lower-status child does not develop the same communication patterns as the middle-class child. This is not to say that he has no speaking skills. The "street culture" of the urban ghetto, for example, is a highly verbal world, and children must become adept with words if they are to function within that culture. After a detailed study of complex verbal patterns used among gangs of adolescent boys in New York City, William Labov concludes:

> Our main finding is that there are a wide variety of verbal skills developed in the Negro Non-Standard English community, which have little connection with the school environment, and which are completely unknown to teachers. Furthermore, many of these skills would be defined as irrelevant to success in the NNE community. (Labov, 1968, p. 1)

The point is that "nonstandard" usage causes harsh reactions from "standard" speakers. The following passage illustrates the problem.

Zoologist Says Dog Yaps Make Sense *

LONDON (EPI)—A zoologist from Oxherd University claims to have deciphered the yelps, snarls, and bays of canines. Dr. Feline, who has been studying dog "speech" for years, says that dogs communicate with each other by means of a very elaborate set of noises, which he has dubbed "fanguage."

. . . Not only are there a great variety of fanguages, but each fanguage has a number of "dogalects" (variations within a fanguage). A hound in one part of a large city, says Dr. Feline, may woof a dogalect which differs in many respects from the dogalect woofed in another part of the city. Curs from these two parts of the city can usually intercommunicate to some extent, but they find it either irritating or amusing. Dr. Feline has observed, moreover, that each mutt acts as though his dogalect were superior to all other dogalects.

Dogalects differ not only among geographical regions, says Dr. Feline, but also between canine classes within a region. The upper-class dogs (consisting of pedigreed animals and those who strive to be like them) woof a different dogalect from the lower-class dogs (consisting of mutts, mongrels, and tramps). For example, the upper-class dogs in London will woof, "Grrr rowlf urr yelp," whereas the lower-class dogs will woof, "Grrr rowlf orr yelp." According to Dr. Feline, this slight difference is enough to cause frothing of the mouth by upper-class and lower-class dogs alike.

* Reprinted by permission from Frank May, *Teaching Language as Communication to Children,* Columbus, Ohio: Merrill, 1967, p. 25.

It is (perhaps unfortunately) very important within speech communities that some usage patterns have high status value while others mark the speaker as inferior. The term "Standard English," like "Bolshevik" (which means majority) and "Great Silent Majority" (a recent variation), is a sham of might-makes-right. The term itself suggests that one usage is better than others. In reality it is only better in some times and places. Like canine speakers of different dogalects, we are all sure that our own usage is correct.

SOME SOLUTIONS

Our solutions, which we shall discuss only in the most general terms, are in the sphere of usage instruction. You will recall that most recommendations in Chapter 9 also focused upon usage. As our main recommendation there was to treat children as people, our main recommendation here is to treat minority children the same way.

If teachers begin to listen closely to the speech of minority-group students, they will learn their usage patterns and discover that their speech is quite intelligible. Because it is intelligible, we need not be so anxious to change it. That does not mean that we need to speak nonstandard to them. They can learn to understand standard usage patterns as easily as we can learn nonstandard. The mix of speech styles in the class, along with the techniques recommended in Chapter 9, will provide ample opportunities to learn about different usage patterns and situations in which each is appropriate. If the classroom contains an ethnic mix of students, there will be ample models to aid learning of many kinds of usage patterns, and little special instruction will be needed. As long as we persist in preventing this ethnic mix, we never will change nonstandard speech patterns, no matter how hard we "teach."

In the past generation, American educators have expended tremendous resources toward the goal of trying to make all children speak like radio announcers. That kind of uniformity is not only impossible to achieve but also undesirable. The method typically used has been instruction in grammar, which is just as unhelpful for remedial purposes as for usual instruction. We suggest the alternative of openly encouraging cultural diversity and working to make each child comfortable within several usage styles. *The major changes must be in attitudes of those of us who teach the children.*

We must face the fact that black English is simply not that different from standard English. Nonstandard speech, say employers, makes black applicants bad risks. But if all blacks started speaking flawless standard tomorrow, it is unlikely that job discrimination would vanish. The real problem is that many whites do not care to be around black faces, no matter how they talk. Again, what we need to change is our attitude—toward nonstandard speech and nonwhite people. Until we make such a change, we will continue to move toward the separate and unequal societies that the Kerner Commission warned us about.

Read This

LABOV, WILLIAM. *The Study of Non-Standard English*. Urbana, Ill.: National Council of Teachers of English, 1970 b.

This readable paperback is a good introduction to the language patterns of nonstandard dialects and to the matrix of social attitudes that surround nonstandard usage.

WILLIAMS, FREDERICK (ed.). *Language and Poverty: Perspectives on a Theme*. Chicago, Ill.: Markham, 1970.

This collection of essays deals with many problems of nonstandard speakers and educational attempts to teach them—essays by many of the top scholars dealing with these problems.

chapter 11

OF CHILDREN AND SPEECH CLINICS, OR "IS MY BABY NORMAL?"

Although this book has been oriented toward discussing normal development, with no attention to the description of abnormal development, the process of normal development has certain implications for those involved in therapy for children with abnormal speech or language. Trying to make an abnormal child more "normal" without knowing about normal children is like trying to glue together a shattered piece of pottery when you do not know what it looked like before it was broken. You are forced to fix something, yet you do not know what it should be like after it is fixed.

This chapter discusses how taking into account the basics of development can aid the clinician in the diagnosis and treatment of language and speech problems.

DIAGNOSIS: EVALUATING SPEECH AND LANGUAGE DEVELOPMENT

At some point, every speech clinician is faced with the task of evaluating a child's language development. Perhaps this is a child referred by the school for "language problems" or a child brought in by his parents because "he doesn't sound right" or "his brother was much further along at his age." Without discussing particular means available to the clinician for conducting this evaluation, we can discuss some of the issues which are involved.

First, the use of the term "evaluate" implies that some comparison will be made between this child's language performance and some ideal performance. Evaluation implies judgment, and you do not judge without some standard. What is the standard against which we evaluate a child's language development? How do you decide whether his development is within normal limits? For many clinicians, the answer to this question lies in the use of standardized tests. A standardized test is one for which performance norms have been collected. That is, the test has been given to a large cross-section of children of different ages, and the performance score of, say, the "average" three-year-old has been gained by averaging the scores of all the three-year-olds who took the test. Although the statistical operations involved may be quite complicated, this is essentially the procedure by which test norms are calculated. Clinicians like to use standardized tests because they can come up with very authoritative statements, such as "This child has a language age of three years six months." This statement can be translated to mean "On this particular test, this child made the same score as the average child aged three years six months."

There are several problems connected with making this kind of statement. First, the statement cannot be applied to language behavior that was not on the test. If the test did not examine the child's ability to use elaborated sentences, then the clinician can make no statement concerning this ability, and he should take care to see that he makes this clear to parents. Beyond this, the clinician may also wish to be careful about making broad statements on the basis of the performance of the "average" child. For most standardized language tests, the norms were collected using white middle-class to upper-middle-class children in northern or midwestern cities. In other words, the language of these children is the ideal against which the language of all children is measured. The moral and esthetic implications of this situation should be obvious. At the very least, if test norms are going to be held up as performance of the average child, then children from many different language environments should be tested when the norms are established. Clinicians should realize that whenever they give a child a standardized language test, they are automatically assuming that the norms for the test are good and appropriate standards for comparison.

When using a language test, whether it is standardized of not, we also assume that the child is giving his best performance. It makes little sense to say: "Now Johnny, I'm going to give you a test, and I don't really care whether you try hard or not. You just say whatever you want to when I ask you a question." On the contrary, we are more likely to say: "Now Johnny, we're going to play a little game, and I want you to think very hard about what I ask, and give me the right answer." The question is: Is our language-testing procedure really designed to tap the best language the child has to offer? Perhaps one example will serve to show the necessity for asking this question. A young clinician went to a local Headstart program to do hearing tests on all the children. The child had to put on a pair of earphones through which he was to hear a tone. When he heard the sound, he was supposed to signal the clinician by saying "now." The clinician had been screening all the city's kindergarten and first-grade children in this way, and she anticipated no problems. However, when she took the first Headstart child out to be tested, he cried and was uncooperative. The second child refused to even put on the earphones, and the third child, although he didn't cry, was so obviously terrified that the clinician decided to try to find out what was going on. After talking with the teacher, and a large group of children, she discovered that some older children had told the group that she was there to give shots. Her strange equipment had done nothing to allay the children's anxiety. After testing the teacher and two aides in front of the class, she was able to test the children without further incident.

This clinician was lucky. She perceived that the children were not behaving normally, and she was able to find out why and alleviate the problem. But think of the ordinary language-testing situation. The clinician is faced with a strange child, one she has never seen before. She does not know what he has been told about why he is being tested, or even whether he has been told that there will be a test. She does not know what his best language performance is, and so she cannot judge whether she is getting that performance from him. She knows that she has another patient in one hour, and besides she has to finish this so the child can go and have his hearing tested.

Now look at this same situation from the child's point of view. He is probably in a strange place with an adult he has never met. He has been taken away from his mother's presence, and does not know what is about to happen. He may be told something about playing a game or answering some questions. Whatever he is told, he realizes immediately that *he doesn't know the rules*. He doesn't know how he is expected to behave. Of all the information he could get, this is most important. But it is this that he is least likely to have.

Remembering that this is a language-testing situation, in which the child is expected to respond in a way that will give the clinician information about his abilities to use his language, let's look at the testing situation as a communication situation. The child is almost certainly unsure of himself—unsure about what is expected of him. He may also be frightened about being alone with a strange adult. What is the logical thing to do when you are frightened and unsure? Anybody with any sense of self-preservation will say and do as little as possible, to avoid the possibility of being wrong. This means minimal communication. It is a rare child who can come off well in a one-to-one situation with a strange adult, and it takes an even rarer child to perform at maximum levels when there is an element of threat in the situation. Yet it is in this situation that we make the assumptions that we are getting the best language performance that child has to offer! It is on the basis of a child's behavior in such a situation that he may be put in a "language enrichment" program or even in a special class.

This brings up another problem involved in evaluating children's language development: The uses that are made of scores on language tests. Many school systems "track" children on the basis of language test scores. That is, children who score low are put in one class and children who score high are put in another. Apart from the questionable rationale for using language test scores to group children, one might ask what is gained by segregating children who have supposedly not developed good language from those who have. Should not the less well-developed children have the benefit of exposure to well-developed language in their peers? Is there justification for our fears that "slow" children will hamper the faster children's learning? The really insidious aspect of all this is that so often a language test score becomes a substitute for an overall estimate of the child's intellectual and communicative abilities in a wide variety of situations. This often results in the horrifying spectacle of a teacher with closed ears looking at a test score and labeling the noisiest kid in the class nonverbal.

Finally, clinicians should know the basics of how speakers of nonstandard dialects sound (see Chapter 10). Often, children speaking nonstandard forms of English are diagnosed as having articulation or language problems. Clinicians should be aware of the fact that tests such as the Goldman-Fristoe Articulation Test, the Peabody Picture Vocabulary Test, and the Illinois Test of Psycholinguistic Ability are biased toward the speech skills of middle-class children. They should also be familiar enough with dialects to tell the difference between dialect-appropriate speech that is different from standard English and errors that need therapy.

This discussion should not be taken to mean that there are no children with language problems. There are many who have obvious difficulty communicating verbally. Their problems may be described as anything from autism to delayed speech; often it is difficult to say exactly what the problem is. There are sensitive and well-trained clinicians who realize the pitfalls involved in the use of standardized tests, and who are searching for some other means of describing the language problems of such children.

Many of these clinicians look to research in communication development of normal children for a firm timetable of what communication behaviors are supposed to occur at what age. Unfortunately, research cannot provide such a timetable. Communication development unfolds at many different rates for different children. In Chapter 2, we reviewed some behaviors that children often perform at certain ages. We repeat the caution we gave there. Do not look too closely at age levels when discussing children's communication behavior. We challenge anyone to come forward with a well-supported, reasonable description of what the "normally developing" child at age three years six months (or any other age) is *supposed* to be doing with language. If research tells us anything at all about this, it tells us that the range of "normal" at any given age is very broad.

Of course, this does not help the clinician who is searching for answers. Some help comes from the fact that the *order* in which communication behaviors emerge is fairly stable. So, for example, if a child is making some distinctions that typically occur at a late stage of development, but missing others that typically appear early, then the missed distinctions probably represent a problem needing clinical help. Further, in most cases there is some correspondence between the speech milestones reported by Lenneberg (see Chapter 2) and motor development milestones. So if a child's motor development is quite mature and his speech sounds very immature, there is likely cause for concern.

Clincians (and parents and teachers) should remember that every child is a dynamic, ever-changing organism. A diagnosis or treatment program undertaken at age three may be totally without basis for the same child at age four. The main lesson from this should be: Keep diagnoses tentative. The patient may change, and having the label of an outgrown disability is a terrible burden for a child to bear.

TREATMENT: CLINICAL TEACHING STRATEGIES

Once a clinician has diagnosed a speech or language problem, his task is to help the child speak normally. In planning teaching strategies for this task, clinicians should keep in mind research findings about how children learn various aspects of communication behavior (see Chapter 8). For example, if the problem were largely syntactic, the teaching approach would be different than if the problem were use of inflectional endings.

Many clinicians base most of their therapy on imitation and reinforcement. These learning strategies are much less powerful than rule-induction or modeling approaches (see Chapter 8). While imitation reinforcement may be highly appropriate for some cases—for example, therapy with severely retarded children

—it may be an inefficient strategy in other cases. You can certainly make any child learn the way rats and animals do (imitation reinforcement), but then you should not be upset if the child then performs little better than such animals. If there is ever to be carryover from language therapy to real-life situations, children must master rule-induction learning strategies.

Two approaches to getting children to learn such strategies may be helpful. First, if Piaget is correct in saying that communication development is only one phase of general cognitive development, training in general cognitive tasks—manipulation of objects, solving puzzles, conservation tasks, and so forth—may sharpen the child's learning strategies to the point at which he can learn to communicate.

At this point, the second approach should come into play. This consists of putting the child in contexts in which he can use language and communication skills to accomplish goals he cares about. Too many clinicians make the therapy situation a lock-step drill session, in which the child uses a particular linguistic form in isolation, over and over again. This approach denies the reality that the therapy situation is also a communication situation and as such can be made a tool for the child's learning. The child should be encouraged to use the full range of his communication skills in the situation—in a way that is meaningful to him. This is, of course, much the same strategy we recommend for teaching normal children in the classroom.

We do not mean to say that all children with communication problems can learn to speak through the methods their normal peers use. We do feel, however, that normal learning strategies should be incorporated into the therapy situation wherever possible.

Neither do we mean to discredit *all* strategies based on operant conditioning or pattern practice. Especially for severely retarded or emotionally disturbed children, these techniques can be effective. But normal or near-normal communication will rarely be taught by these methods alone. To master the complexities of language, more powerful learning tools are necessary, and this learning is more likely to occur in more realistic communication situations.

BIBLIOGRAPHY

ALLAND, ALEXANDER. *Evolution and Human Behavior.* New York: Natural History Press, 1967.

AUER, J. JEFFERY, and EDWARD B. JENKINSON (eds.). *On Teaching Speech in Elementary and Junior High Schools.* Bloomington, Ill.: Indiana University Press, 1971.

BATES, REED. A Study in the Acquisition of Language. Unpublished Ph.D. dissertation. University of Texas, 1967.

BEVER, THOMAS. "The Cognitive Basis for Linguistic Structures," in John R. Hayes (ed.), *Cognition and the Development of Language.* New York: Wiley, 1970.

BLOOM, LOIS. "Why Not Pivot Grammars?" *Journal of Speech and Hearing Disorders,* 36 (Feb. 1971), 40–50.

BROWN, ROGER. *Words and Things.* New York: Free Press, 1958.

BROWN, ROGER. *Psycholinguistics.* New York: Free Press, 1970.

BROWN, ROGER, and URSULA BELLUGI. "Three Processes in the Child's Acquisition of Syntax," *Harvard Educational Review,* 34 (1964), 133–151.

BROWN, ROGER, COURTNEY CAZDEN, and URSULA BELLUGI. "The Child's Grammar from I to III," in John Hill (ed.), *1967 Minnesota Symposia on Child Psychology.* Minneapolis: University of Minnesota Press, 1969.

BROWN, ROGER, and C. HANLON. "Derivational Complexity and Order of Acquisition in Child Speech," in John R. Hayes (ed.), *Cognition and the Development of Language.* New York: Wiley, 1970.

CAZDEN, COURTNEY. Environmental Assistance to the Child's Acquisition of Grammar. Unpublished Ph.D. dissertation. Harvard University, Graduate School of Education, 1965.

CAZDEN, COURTNEY. "The Neglected Situation in Child Language Research and Education," in Frederick Williams (ed.), *Language and Poverty.* Chicago: Markham, 1970.

CHOMSKY, CAROL. *The Acquisition of Syntax in Children from 5 to 10.* Cambridge, Mass.: MIT Press, 1969.

CHOMSKY, NOAM. *Language and Mind.* New York: Harcourt Brace Jovanovich, 1968.

CHOMSKY, NOAM, and MORRIS HALLE. *The Sound Pattern of English.* New York: Harper & Row, 1968.

DALE, PHILIP. *Language Development: Structure and Function.* New York: Dryden Press, 1972.

DEESE, JAMES. *Psycholinguistics.* Boston: Allyn & Bacon, 1970.

ERVIN, SUSAN. "Imitation and Structural Change in Children's Language," in Eric Lenneberg (ed.), *New Directions in the Study of Language.* Cambridge, Mass.: MIT Press, 1964.

FLAVELL, JOHN. *Communication and the Development of Role-Taking Skills in Children.* New York: Wiley, 1968.

FRANKE, CARL. "Uber die erste Laustufe der Kinder," *Anthropos* (1912), 663–676.

FURTH, HANS. *Piaget and Knowledge.* Englewood Cliffs, N.J.: Prentice-Hall, 1969.

FURTH, HANS G. *Piaget for Teachers.* Englewood Cliffs, N.J.: Prentice-Hall, 1972.

GARDNER, R. A., and BEATRICE GARDNER. "Teaching Sign Language to a Chimpanzee," *Science* 165 (1969), 664–672.

HOLT, JOHN. *How Children Learn.* New York: Pitman, 1967.

HOPPER, ROBERT. "Communicative Development and Children's Responses to Questions," *Speech Monographs,* XXXVIII (1971), 1–9.

HOPPER, ROBERT. "Expanding the Notion of Competence," *The Speech Teacher,* XX (January 1971), 29–35.

HYMES, DELL. *On Communicative Competence.* Philadelphia: University of Pennsylvania Press, 1970.

HYMES, DELL. "Linguistic Theory and the Functions of Speech." Prepared for International Days in Sociolinguistics, Rome, Italy, Sept., 1969.

JAKOBSON, ROMAN, and MORRIS HALLE. *Fundamentals of Language.* The Hague: Mouton, 1956.

KESSEL, F. The Development of Children's Comprehension from 6 to 12. Unpublished Ph.D. dissertation. University of Minnesota, 1969.

KLIMA, EDWARD S., and URSULA BELLUGI. "Syntactic Regularities in the Speech of Children," in J. Lyons and R. Wales (eds.), *Psycholinguistics Papers.* Edinburgh: Edinburgh University Press, 1966.

LABOV, WILLIAM. "The Logic of Nonstandard English," in Frederick Williams (ed.), *Language and Poverty.* Chicago: Markham, 1970a.

LABOV, WILLIAM. *The Study of Nonstandard English*. Urbana, Ill.: National Council of Teachers of English, 1970b.

LABOV, WILLIAM, and others. *A Study of the Nonstandard English used by Negro and Puerto Rican Speakers in New York City*. Final report, U.S. Office of Education Cooperative Research Project No. 3288, 1968.

LENNEBERG, ERIC. "The Natural History of Language," in F. Smith and G. Miller (eds.), *The Genesis of Language*. Cambridge, Mass.: MIT Press, 1966.

LENNEBERG, ERIC. *Biological Foundations of Language*. New York: Wiley, 1967.

LEWIS, M. M. *Language, Thought and Personality in Infancy and Childhood*. New York: Basic Books, 1963.

MAY, FRANK. *Teaching Language as Communication to Children*. Columbus, Ohio: Merrill, 1967.

MCNEILL, DAVID. Development of the Semantic System. Unpublished paper. Harvard University, Center for Cognitive Studies, 1965.

MCNEILL, DAVID. "Developmental Psycholinguistics," in Frank Smith and George Miller (eds.), *The Genesis of Language*. Cambridge, Mass.: MIT Press, 1966.

MCNEILL, DAVID. *The Acquisition of Language*. New York: Harper & Row, 1970.

MEHLER, J., and T. BEVER. "Cognitive Capacity of Very Young Children," *Science,* 161 (October 1967), 141–142.

MOFFETT, JAMES. *Teaching the Universe of Discourse*. New York: Houghton Mifflin, 1968.

PIAGET, JEAN. *The Child's Conception of the World,* trans. Marjorie Wordon. New York: Harcourt Brace Jovanovich, 1928.

POSTMAN, NEIL, and CHARLES WEINGARTNER. *Teaching as a Subversive Activity*. New York: Delacorte, 1969.

PREMACK, D. "Language in Chimpanzees?" *Science,* 169 (May 1971), 808–822.

PULASKI, MARY ANN SPENCER. *Understanding Piaget*. New York: Harper & Row, 1971.

QUINE, WILLARD. "Speaking of Objects," in J. Fodor and J. Katz (eds.), *The Structure of Language*. Englewood Cliffs, N.J.: Prentice-Hall, 1964.

SALUS, PETER. *Linguistics*. New York: Bobbs-Merrill, 1969.

SILBERMAN, CHARLES. *Crisis in the Classroom*. New York: Random House, 1970.

SINCLAIR-DE-ZWART, HERMINA. "Developmental Psycholinguistics," in D.

Elkind and J. Flavell (eds.), *Studies in Cognitive Development.* New York: Oxford University Press, 1969.

SKINNER, B. F. *Verbal Behavior.* New York: Appleton, 1957.

SLOBIN, D. I. "The Acquisition of Russian as a Native Language," in F. Smith and G. Miller (eds.), *The Genesis of Language.* Cambridge, Mass.: MIT Press, 1966.

SLOBIN, D. I. *Psycholinguistics.* Glenview, Ill.: Scott, Foresman, 1971.

U.S. Riot Commission. Report of the National Advisory Commission on Civil Disorders. New York: Bantam Books, 1968. (Kerner Commission)

WHORF, BENJAMIN. *Language, Thought and Reality.* Cambridge, Mass.: MIT Press, 1956.

WILLIAMS, FREDERICK (ed.). *Language and Poverty.* Chicago: Markham, 1970.

WILLIAMS, FREDERICK, and RITA C. NAREMORE. "On the Functional Analysis of Social Class Differences in Modes of Speech," *Speech Monographs* 36 (June 1969), 77–102.

INDEX